ADVANCES IN BIOMEDICAL EXPERIMENTAL TECHNIQUES IN PHARMACOLOGICAL ASSAYS

by

Archana R. Juvekar

M. Pharm, Ph.D (Tech)

Professor in Pharmacology & Physiology
Department of Pharmaceutical Sciences & Technology,
Institute of Chemical Technology,
(University under Section 3 of UGC Act 1956;
Maharashtra Government's "Elite Status and Center of Excellence"
Formerly UDCT/UICT, University of Mumbai)
Nathalal Parekh Marg, Matunga, Mumbai - 411 019.

S. R. Naik

M.Sc. (Biochemistry), Ph.D. (Pharmacology)

Emiretus Professor,
Dr. D.Y. Patil Institute of Pharmaceutical Sciences and Research Center,
Pune - 411018.

Ex. General Manager (R&D, QCL and QA), Hindustan Antibiotics Ltd.
Pune - 411018.

Ex Professor and Principal, Prin. K. M. Kundnani College of Pharmacy,
Mumbai - 400 005.

Professor and Principal of Institute of Pharmacutical Sciences,
Lonavala, Pune.

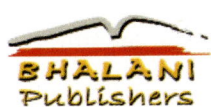

BHALANI
Publishers

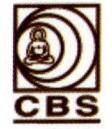

CBS

CBS PUBLISHERS & DISTRIBUTORS PVT. LTD.

W0080619

© *Bhalani Publishers*

First Edition : 2018

ISBN No. 978-93-83794-04-1

PUBLISHED BY :

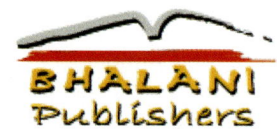

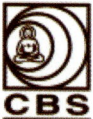

Rajesh Bhalani for
BHALANI PUBLISHERS
1201, Avanti Building, Neelkanth Kingdom,
Vidyavihar (W), Mumbai - 400086.
Mob: +91 9867214519
E-mail : bhalanipublishers@gmail.com

Satish Kumar Jain for
CBS PUBLISHERS & DISTRIBUTORS PVT. LTD.
4819/XI Prahlad Street, 24 Ansari Road,
Daryaganj,
New Delhi - 110002, India.
Ph.: 011-23289259, 23266861/67 Fax: 23243014
✉: delhi@cbspd.com/cbspubs@airtelmail.in
Website: www.cbspd.com

Corporate Office: 204 FIE, Industrial Area,
Patparganj, Delhi - 110092
Ph.: 49344934, Fax: 49344935
✉: publishing@cbspd.com

PRINTED & BOUND BY :

ASHISH ARTS - Mumbai.
✉: bharat.ashisharts@gmail.com

EDITORS & CONTRIBUTORS

EDITORS

Prof. Archana R. Juvekar   Prof. S. R. Naik

CONTRIBUTORS

Prof. S. R. Naik

Snehal N. Mestry
(ICT, Mumbai)

Malvika S. Gursahani
(ICT, Mumbai)

Shilpee G. Chanda
(ICT, Mumbai)

Prof. Deepti D. Bandawane
(P.E. Society's Modern College of Pharmacy, Nigdi, Pune)

Dr. Mrinal M. Sanaye
(Prin. K. M. K College of Pharmacy, Mumbai)

Prof. Archana R. Juvekar

Sarayu A. Pai
(ICT, Mumbai)

Pratibha A. Daroi
(ICT, Mumbai)

Jyoti S. Batgire
(ICT, Mumbai)

Abhijit S. Mali
(Ajanta Pharmaceuticals, Mumbai)

Komal S. Gupta
(Bhavans' College, Mumbai)

PREFACE

The book entitled "Advances in Biomedical Experimental Techniques in Pharmacological Assays" has been written with a view to facilitate the understanding of the fundamental aspects of the screening methodologies used in drug discovery. Screening of potential molecules in animal models is one of the most crucial phases in drug discovery and development which helps to identify potential leads which can be taken up for further studies. This book provides a lucid understanding of the subject with the help of illustrations. The book has been written to cater to the needs of post-graduate students from the fields of medicine, pharmaceutical sciences and life sciences including biomedical sciences.

The topics included in the book have been selected carefully considering the syllabus of medicine, pharmaceutical sciences, life sciences and biomedical sciences. This textbook attempts to bring forth the pressing need of the hour to emphasize the importance of new generation and the state-of-art techniques in drug screening pertaining to drug discovery and drug development, including new approaches in respective chapters. The book has been edited on the basis of the editors' vast and in depth experience in drug research of over 30 years.

The book comprises screening methods for drugs acting on the central nervous system, autonomic nervous system and renal system. Anti-inflammatory, analgesic, anti-arthritic drugs, anti-diabetic, anti-hyperlipidemic, hepato-protectives, anti-asthmatics and antioxidants. Apart from these, in order to provide a holistic understanding of the drug discovery process, chapters on toxicological techniques and statistical methods of analysis are covered.

Editors are confident that this book would certainly provide latest information in drug screening processes, in drug discovery and would prove of immense help to postgraduates and doctoral students.

FOREWORD

Exponential progress in human biological research and development is based on the fact that methods in drug discovery have rapidly developed in the recent past. For future pharmacists and bio-scientists it is essential to be familiarized in their early education with both traditional pharmacological methods as well as recent developments and approaches in this field.

The present first edition of this book particularly addresses this need. After introducing the central nervous system through the foundations of experimental methods in various applications, the editors demonstrate the importance of screening methods for the discovery of molecules with a therapeutic and diagnostic potential.

The scope of the detailed screening methods, for a reliable discovery of pharmacological effects of potential drugs, includes detection of hepatoprotective activity, antihyperglycemic, antihyperlipidemic, antioxidant agents so on and so forth.

The book is complemented by a comprehensive introduction on toxicological methods and techniques, as well as statistical basics, relevant to experimental pharmacological research.

The editors have succeeded in demonstrating the importance of knowledge related to screening methods, for anyone involved in drug discovery/development. Their way to accompany screening methods, by knowledge of experimental methods at the beginning and statistical know-how in the end works well and provides an excellent all in one textbook for students of pharmaceutical and biomedical sciences and related study programs as well as for young scientists in the field.

Prof. Dr. Gerhard Fortwengel,
University of Applied Sciences and Arts,
MPH, Hochschule Hannover,
Germany

FOREWORD

Use of animals in biomedical research has contributed to the advancement of knowledge, unfolding of many physiological phenomena, understanding of disease pathophysiology and development of new drugs. Though in the recent times several attempts have been made to develop alternatives to animal experimentation, they fail to replace the experiments on the animals completely. The alternatives can be used for demonstration of certain phenomena or to learn basic skills, mainly to save lives or suffering of animals, which are otherwise used for these purpose. To some extent such alternatives are used in early stages of drug discovery or development but here too animal experimentation provide better predictability of efficacy and safety of drugs. This is because animals share many basic physiological and pathological processes of humans. Hence for scientific studies, essential use of animals is justified, albeit ensuring 3 R principles-Replacement, Reduction and Refinement.

Unfortunately, in many institutions a tendency has been observed to avoid use of animals. This has stemmed from wrong concepts and moves regarding the animal experimentation, inadequate resources for maintenance of animal house environment and inertia of the faculty and administrators to take requisite efforts for the same. As a result there is limited or almost no training offered in educational institutions in relevant laboratory skills of animal handling or classical pharmacological assays using them. We are thus missing out an important mile stone in biomedical research.

Barring one or two textbooks, which are out of reach of students as well as faculty, we do not have any standard book or electronic database to refer to. Most of the researchers look for the methodologies published in journals which are not explicitly narrated and spend more time and man hours in standardization in their own laboratories. The intricacies in these methodologies are hardly shared.

In such a grim scenario, the book, "Advances in Biomedical Experimental Techniques in Pharmacological Assays" has emerged as a ray of hope. The writings in this book are the distillates of long standing experience and expertise of the two eminent pharmacologists, Dr. Archana Juvekar and Dr. S. R. Naik in the field of animal experimentation required for drug discovery and development. Both of them have presented before the readers a wide range of classical techniques which are in use for perhaps more than a century as well as those which have been developed recently taking advantage of technological advances.

The book covers the most commonly used screening methods pertaining to evaluation of drugs acting on CNS, ANS and renal system. Whenever necessary, the chapter includes techniques used for tissues, which belong to the same system but having different properties e.g. Chapter 3 presents techniques used for drugs acting on smooth muscles, cardiac muscles and skeletal muscles. In addition, pharmacological assays detecting hepatoprotective, anti-hyperglycemic, anti-hyperlipidaemic, anti-Inflammatory, anti-arthritic and analgesic, anti-asthmatic and antioxidant potential of drugs have been selected for inclusion. It also provides information about the latest assays done using genetically engineered animals as in Chapter 5. Not only efficacy testing, but the book covers toxicological methods and techniques in a separate chapter. Both, *in-vitro* and *in-vivo* techniques have been elaborated making it a complete evaluation profile for drug under the test. A chapter on 'Statistical methods in experimental pharmacological research' is an important inclusion. Sound statistical background helps each and every stage of research, starting from deciding research design and planning to presentation, analysis and interpretation of data.

Each of the chapter is written in a simple, lucid style which is easy to comprehend. The boxes, tables and diagrams highlight the key points and provide guidance to experimental design. An attempt has been made to provide details of animal models, various insults, mechanism of their actions and variables to be tested. Wherever appropriate, purpose and principles of assays have been elaborated in details. It is a treat for any researcher to have all these assays compiled at one place. The references add flavor to this treat. The references are recent, many from 2000 onwards and can compel the interested readers to visit to the original articles.

This book provides an opportunity to postgraduate students of pharmacology, pharmacy, biomedical sciences to get familiarized with the world of animal experimental techniques. It will make them think about what they should do for their own research question and will enable them to foresee what may happen if they undertake a particular study. More the time researchers spend on careful selection and planning of their experimental technique, more is the guarantee of successful evaluation.

In a nutshell, this book is a 'must read' book for a researcher venturing into drug discovery and development. I congratulate both the editors and the publisher of the book for their praiseworthy efforts.

Dr. Nirmala Rege
Professor and Head,
Department of Pharmacology and Therapeutics,
Seth GS Medical College and KEM Hospital,
Mumbai- 400 012.

ACKNOWLEDGEMENT

I always thought that the acknowledgement's page was something every editor/author put in because it was sort of a necessity in every book. It is only when I got around to writing this book, did I realise how much help so many people were to me. Without these people, this book could well have been another pipe dream. I now realise that the acknowledgement is something that really comes from the bottom of the heart of every writer.

If I were to thank only one individual, it would be my senior colleague and co-editor of this book Prof. S. R. Naik. His patience, knowledgeable direction and sustained interest culminated in the completion of this book. I express my sincere gratitude to Vice Chancellor Prof. G. D. Yadav and Prof. Mariam Degani, Head, Pharmaceutical Sciences and Technology for their continuous support and encouragement.

I am fortunate to have a team of postgraduates like Dr. Deepti Bandawane, Miss. Malvika S. Gursahani, Miss. Snehal N. Mestry, Miss. Sarayu A. Pai, Mrs. Pratibha A. Daroi, Miss. Shilpee G. Chanda, Miss. Jyoti S. Batgire, Dr. Nitin B. Gawali, Dr. Mrinal M. Sanaye and Ms. Komal S. Gupta who have contributed chapters and co-operated from time to time, in my seemingly arduous goal.

I am deeply grateful to my dear friends Prof. K. S. Laddha and Prof. Vandana B. Patravale for their guidance and support in motivating me and made my journey memorable. I would also like to extend my heartful thanks to Dr. Ajit Kumar, Dr. Sanjeev Nimbkar, Mr. Daka Krishna Reddy and Miss. Padmini Deshpande who have helped me selflessly.

I would like to express my deepest gratitude to my family for their continuous support and encouragement in my endeavours.

My special thanks to the Publishers, Mr. Rajesh Bhalani of Bhalani Publishers, printer - Mr. Bharat Shah and his team Mrs. Neeta Sakpal of Ashish Arts for their comprehensive involvement and unstinted support in the completion of the project.

Above all the unseen "Hand of God" propelled this effort to fruition.

Dr. Archana Juvekar
M. Pharm, Ph.D (Tech)

CONTENTS

ABBREVIATION

$1O_2$	: Singlet Oxygen 2,4-DNPH:2, 4-dinitrophenylhydrazine		EEG	: Electroencephalogram
5HIAA	: 5-Hydroxy Indole Acetic Acid		FDA	: Food and Drugs Administration
5-HT	: 5-Hydroxy Tryptamine		Fe	: Iron
6OHDM	: 6-Hydroxy Dopamine		FEV1	: Forced Expiratory Volume
AC	: Atherogenic Coefficient		FRAP	: Ferric Reducing Antioxidant Power
AI	: Atherosclerosis Index		FVC	: Forced Vital Capacity
ABTS	: 2,2'-azinobis-3-hylbenzothiazo-line-6-sulfonic acid		G-6-PDH	: Glucose-6-phosphate dehydrogenase
ACh	: Acetylcholine		GABA	: Gamma-aminobutyric Acid
ADP	: Adenine diphosphatase		GLUT	: Glucose Transporter
ALP	: Alkaline Phosphatase		GPI	: Glucose-6 phosphate isomerase
ALT	: Alanine Aminotransferase		GPx/GPOX	: Glutathione peroxidase
ANS	: Autonomic Nervous System		GR	: Glutathione reductase
As	: Arsenic		GSH	: Reduced glutathione
AST	: Aspartate Aminotransferase		GSSG	: Glutathione, Oxidized Form
ATP	: Adenosine Triphosphate		GST	: Glutathione transferase
BAG1	: BCl-2 associated athanogene 1		H&E	: Hematoxylin and Eosin
BCl-2	: B-cell lymphoma2		H_2O_2	: Hydrogen Peroxide
BDNF	: Brain Derived - Neurotrophic Factor		HDL-C	: High-density Lipoprotein - Cholesterol
BHT	: Butylated Hydroxy Toluene		Hg	: Mercury
BSA	: Bovine Serum Albumin		HMG-CoA	: 3-hydroxy-3-methylglutaryl-CoA
CAT	: Catalase		HNO_2	: Nitrous Acid
Cd	: Cadmium		HOCl	: Hypochlorous Acid
CDNB	: 1-chloro-2,4-dinitrobenzene		HPA	: Hypothalamic-Pituitary-Adrenal axis
CHE	: Cholesterol esterases		HPRT	: Hypoxanthine - Phosphoribosyltransferase
CHO	: Cholesterol oxidase		IC_{50}	: Concentration of the compound - causing 50% inhibition
CNS	: Central Nervous System		ICH	: International Conference on - Harmonization
CRR	: Cardiac Risk Ratio		IDDM	: Insulin-dependent Diabetes Mellitus
CVD	: Cardiovascular Disease		IDPN	: β, β-iminodipropionitrile
DA	: Dopamine		IL	: Interleukin
DNA	: Deoxynucleic Acid		IL-1Ra	: IL-1 Receptor Antagonist
DOPAC	: 4-hydroxyphenylacetic acid		INH	: Isonicotonic Acid Hydrazide
DPPH	: 1,1-diphenyl-2-picrylhydrazyl		LA	: Linoleic Acid
DTH	: Delayed Type Hypersensitivity		LDL-C	: Low-density Lipoprotein Cholesterol
DTNB	: 5,5'-dithiobis(2-nitrobenzoic acid)		LHT	: Learned Helplessness Test
EA	: Egg Albumin		LOAEL	: Lowest Observed Adverse Effect - Level

LOO•	: Lipid Peroxyl Radical		PMS	: Phenazine Methosulphate
LOOH	: Lipid Peroxide		pO_2	: Partial Pressure of Oxygen
LTD_4	: Leukotriene		PPARα	: Peroxisome Proliferator-activated Receptor Alpha
LVPD	: Left Ventricular Pressure - Development		PSS	: Physiological Salt Solution
MAO	: Monoamine Oxidase		REM	: Rapid Eye Movement
MDA	: Malondialdehyde		RNS	: Reactive Nitrogen Species
MF	: Microfilament		ROO•	: Peroxyl Radical
MRI	: Magnetic Resonance Imaging		ROS	: Reactive Oxygen Species
N_2O_3	: Dinitrogen Trioxide		SDStr	: Social Defeat Stress
NAPQI	: N-acetyl-p-benzoquinone		SDS	: Sodium Dodecyl Sulfate
NBT	: Nitro Blue Tetrazolium		SL	: Sarcolemma
NE	: Norepinephrine		SOD	: Superoxide Dismutase
NIDDM	: Non-insulin-dependent - Diabetes Mellitus		SR	: Sarcoplasmic Reticulum
NO	: Nitric Oxide		β-NADP	: β-Nicotinamide Adenine - Dinucleotide Phosphate-Oxidized Form
NO•	: Nitric Oxide Radical			
NO_2•	: Nitrogen Dioxide Radical		β-NADPH	: β-Nicotinamide Adenine - Dinucleotide Phosphate-Reduced Form
NOAEL	: No-observed Adverse Effect Level			
NSAID	: Non-Steroidal Anti-inflammatory - Drug			
O_2•⁻	: Superoxide Radical		STZ	: Streptozotocin
O_3	: Ozone		TBA	: Thiobarbituric Acid
OECD	: Organization for Economic - Co-operation and Development		TBARS	: Thiobarbituric Acid Reactive - Substances
OH•	: Hydroxyl Radical		TC	: Total Cholesterol
ONOO⁻	: Peroxynitrite		TCA	: Trichloroacetic Acid
ORAC	: Oxygen Radical - Absorbance Capacity		TE	: Trolox Equivalent
			TFA	: Trifluoroacetic Acid
P407	: Poloxamer 407		TG	: Triglyceride
PARP	: Poly(ADP-ribose) Polymerase		TMM	: Tetramethyl Murexide - Ammonium
PAS	: Periodic Acid Schiff			
Pb	: Lead		TNB	: 5-thio (2-nitrobenzoic acid)
PBS	: Phosphate Buffer Saline		TPTZ	: 2,4,6-tripyridyl-s-triazine
PCA	: Passive Cutaneous Anaphylaxis		trkB	: Tropomyosin related kinase B
pCO_2	: Partial Pressure of Carbon dioxide		TST	: Tail Suspension Test
PEFR	: Peak Expiratory Flow Rate		UR	: Unconditioned Response
PET	: Positron Emission Tomography		V_2	: Vasopressin -2
PG	: Proteoglycans		VLA_4	: Very Late Antigen-4
PGF-2α	: Prostaglandin F-2α		WHO	: World Health Organization

1 GENERAL INTRODUCTION TO CENTRAL NERVOUS SYSTEM

CENTRAL NERVOUS SYSTEM AND CNS DRUG SCREENING

This chapter mainly covers the methods used in evaluating the effects of drugs on the CNS. The functions of the CNS are extremely complex and widespread. Therefore one can attempt at his best to present very sketchy account of the techniques used to evaluate the effects of drugs/agents on some of the functions of CNS. The **Fig. 1.1a** represents frontal view and **Fig. 1.1b** represents the lateral view of the typical human brain structure.

Many of the essential biochemical connections of the nerve cells are dependent upon several morphological features: synaptic contact is mediated by chemical molecules "neurotransmitters" which ensures the continued propagation of electric impulses through several sequential units of the system of chemical neurotransmission that brings out changes in the cation distribution. Further, while the energy utilizing mechanisms, which depends on their redistribution and are not specific to the nervous system, but they have specific relevant importance to the nervous system.

Nerve cells have unique property and ability to trigger off and to maintain conduction of electrical impulses over long distances without significant loss of strength of the conducted impulse. However, their specific connection is not only with nerve cells but also non-neural largest cells such as the endocrinological glands and muscles.

One aspect of the biochemical function of the brain can be reflected in the efficient production of energy, essential to the unique process of brain activity as well as its function.

Brain depends for its ability to function normally on a constant supply of glucose and oxygen from the blood stream, because it has virtually no reserves for chemical

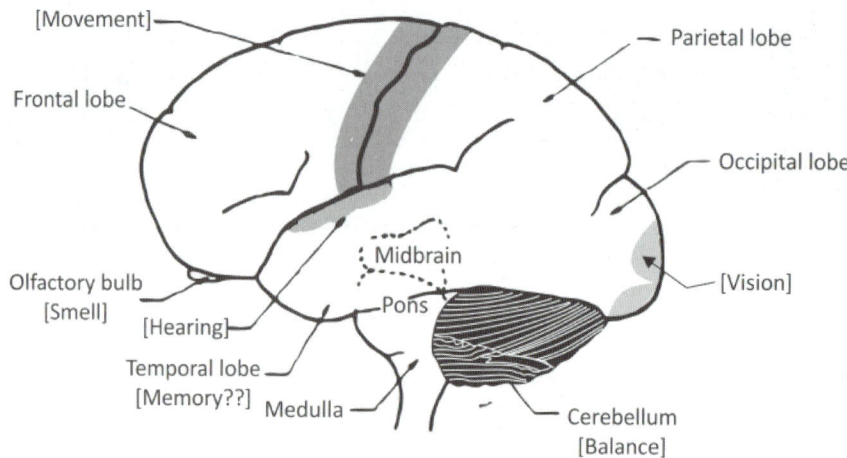

Fig. 1.1a: Human brain.

energy, compared with other peripheral tissues or organs. It must be emphasized that the high sensitivity to any impairment in the normal process of energy metabolism is likely to impair the consequences of mental function. It is largely seen in children who have serious deficiency in the metabolic process that results in impaired mental function (mental retardation).

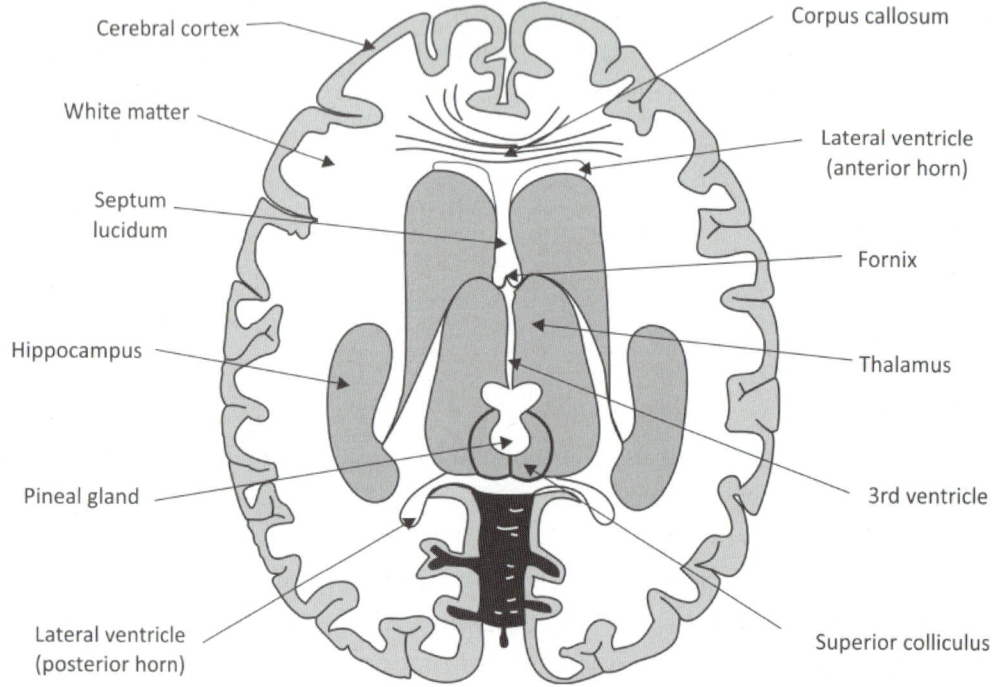

Fig. 1.1b: Lateral view of human brain.

Table 1.1: Enumerates the various parts of the brain and their functional role

Part	Functional role
Cerebral cortex	Motor, special sensory function also involved in attention, memory consciousness and abstract thoughts
Limbic system	Integrates emotions with motor and visceral activities
Hippocampus	Recent memory and memory loss
Hypothalamus	Regulates emotion, integrates a number of autonomic functions, involves cardiovascular, neuroendocrine systems and temperature regulation, eating, drinking and sexual behavior
Brain stem: (medulla, pons, midbrain etc)	Houses reticular activation responsible for sleep and a wakefulness. Stimulation of electrical response, induce arousal.
Cerebellum	An important structure responsible for maintenance of posture and can be affected by many drugs
Spinal cord	Responsible for motor, sensory and autonomic functions are affected by CNS stimulants (strychnine), general anaesthetics and narcotic analgesia.

MACROSCOPIC APPEARANCE:

The observations of cell bodies, axons, dendrites and dendritic spines are made using light microscope, which lead to the 'neuronal hypothesis' with synaptic junctions. Subsequently, the fine structure of synapses were demonstrated by light microscopy. The occurrence of variety of all types are divided into two main groups: the neurons (excitable nerve cells) and glial (non-excitable cells).

NEURONS:

Neurons may have large or small cell bodies (perikarya) possessing a large nucleus containing a prominent nucleolus, a high content ribosome in the cytoplasm and high content of mitochondria. These characteristic features are compatible with active synthetic and secretary activities and the large capacity for energy production **(Fig. 1.2)**. Essential characteristics are the major processes which form extensions of the outer cell membrane: axons and dendrites.

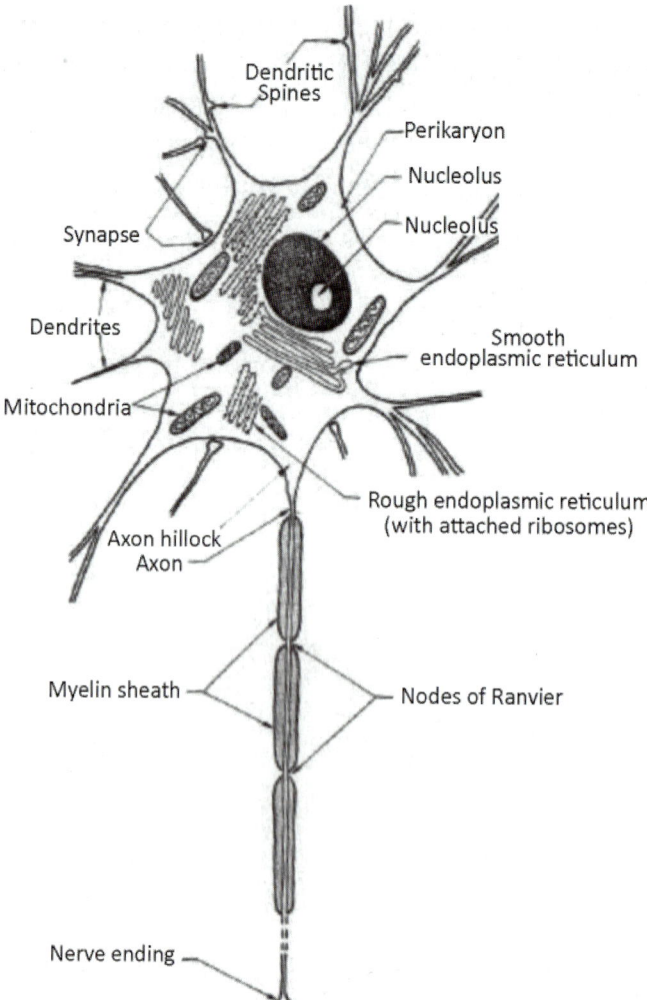

Fig. 1.2: Parts of neuron.

The axons covered by myelin sheath are made up of spiral membrane (giving impression of concentric rings in cross section) which form the electrical impulse from the efferent neurons to another part of the system, and all connections are made through synapses. Whereas dendrites are usually thicker, shorter and highly branched, and do not have a myelin sheath which normally carry the transmission from the synapse to afferent nerve cells.

The major types of cell are identified largely by means of their processes- unipolar (cells containing one axon, ex. sensory cells of ganglia), "bipolar" (cells having two processes, an axon and a dendrite) which are largely distributed in the granular layer of cerebellum. Whereas sensory receptor cells are concerned with sight, smell and hearing. Most neurons are multipolar-containing one axon and many dendrites. Multipolar cells fall into two categories-pyramidal cells and stellate cells.

GLIAL CELLS:

These cells are non excitable, smaller but also have an intrinsic ability of generating the process from their cell bodies. These processes are relatively short and often highly branched. The 3 main types of astrocytes; often found close to blood vessels which makes contact with blood capillary wall and largely concerned with nutrition and acting as mediators in the transport of materials to the neurons. Oligodendroglia is also stellate cells and is concerned with the myelin sheath of axons, produced by them. Schwann cells which perform the same function in myelination of peripheral nerves outside the brain.

SYNAPSE:

The junction of one nerve cell with another nerve with innervated target cells such as in muscle or endocrine glands or the axon approaches its point of contact with the subsequent or post-synaptic structure, known as the nerve ending. In some exceptional cases presynaptic and post synaptic membranes are fused and are called as electrical synapse. They are also known as electrical coupling between the neurons.

The communication between neurons in the CNS occurs through chemical synapses in majority of the cases. The traditional view of the synapse is that it functions like a valve, transmitting information in one direction. At present it is clear that the synapse can generate signals that feedback into synaptic terminal to modify transmitter release. The major neurotransmitters are briefly described below. Large number of small molecules have been isolated from the brain tissues and studied using variety of approaches,methods, systems and demonstrated as neurotransmitters. They are described briefly below:

Some important properties of neurotransmitters:

- The chemical substances must reside in the nerve endings(pre-synaptic terminal pathway) and should have discrete rather than a uniform pattern of distribution.

- It must be originated within neurons and released from the presynaptic nerve terminal (demonstrated by biochemical analysis and immuno-cytochemical techniques especially for enzymes and peptides).

- Local concentration of the substance should be proportionally related to the function of neuronal structure and variations in its concentration should take place in response to functional alterations in the neuron(s).

- When it acts on or applied post-synaptic cell body, the chemical substance may mimic the action of the synapticallly released chemical transmitter.

- Blocking agents of such chemical substance should elicit effects by blocking/preventing the access of the transmitter to the specific receptor sites.

- The neuromodulatory effect has been defined to denote a neuronally released mediator; the effects of such chemicals do not conform to those of neurotransmitters. Such chemicals cover neuronal peptide mediators, which normally acts slowly and also remotely from where it is released includes also nitric oxide (gas) and arachidonic acid breakdown products that are not stored or released like conventional neurotransmitters, and these may originate from non-neuronal cells as well as neuronal cells.

- The established central neurotransmitters have been isolated from the brain tissue using a variety of methods, techniques and other approaches. The neurotransmitters pharmacologically active are: acetylcholine (ACh), dopamine (DA). Amino acids like gamma aminobutyric acid (GABA), glutamine, aspartate and glycine. Amines like 5-hydroxytryptamine (5-HT), nor-epinehrine (NE), histamine, opiod peptides, tachkinins and endocannabinoids.

- With such background information I shall describe various evaluation methods, as some call it screening methods for drugs acting on Central Nervous system. This include some specific tests for specialized activities.

- All these methodologies or techniques are simple and can be carried out in most of the pharmacology laboratories of academic institutions (pharmaceutical sciences, medical colleges or any biomedical institutions).

- Highly sophisticated techniques involving use of precision electronic gadgets or equipments have not been mentioned as it would be difficult to perform in most of the institutions.

2 EXPERIMENTAL METHODS IN CNS PHARMACOLOGY

General screening are performed in experimental animals (mice, rats and others), and that include carefully recording various behavioural output (clinical symptoms) after the administration of test compounds, such as onset, duration, and peak effects on various systems (e.g. CNS, CVS, ANS) using suitable behavioural parameters, toxic reactions, mortality and cause of death.

The well planned primary screening largely helps to understand pharmacodynamic and pharmacokinetic aspects such as absorption and distribution including process of drug kinetic pattern (peak hour of effect and duration effect, approximate LD_{50} value) including vital physiological parameters associated with drug effects. Keeping in mind above mentioned aspects the proper protocol or behaviour output recording sheet can be designed by including specific or characteristic clinical symptoms related to various organ systems of the body (refer the proto-type recording sheet – **Table 2.1a & 2.1b**). The observed pharmacological effects can be scored using suitable scale following administration of different doses of test drug.

A prototype observation sheet enclosed enumerate varied type of vital clinical symptoms such as decreased motor activity, loss of muscle tone, motor in-coordination, posture, miosis and mydriasis (size of pupil), others such as pinna reflex, corneal reflex, righting reflex, placing reflex, hypnosis, catatonia (characteristic effect of rigidity), catalepsy (characteristic effect of immobility associated with ptosis), explorative activities, convulsions, stupor, hyperactivity, aggressiveness, diuresis, defecation, sweating, salivation and many more). It is also possible to measure analgesia and record body temperature during observation. Careful and well directed behavioural studies may provide information on pharmacological profile of test substance, including approximate LD_{50}.

After primary pharmacological screening, one can undertake the detailed investigation by applying specific screening methods or tests using either 1/10th or

Table 2.1a: Prototype observation sheet for rodents

Approximately LD_{50} _____ mg/kg i.p. mice   Cause of depth _____

_____

PRIMARY SCREENING

Code ____ = no effect

+ + = Strong effect   + = Mild effect

GROSS OBSERVATION (MICE)	DOSE MG/KG	REF-			CARDIOVASCULAR (DOGS OR CATS)			
		−	+	++		−	+	++
Stimulant					Adrenergic			
Hyperactivity					Adrenergic Blockade			
Irritability					Cholinergic			
Tremor					Anticholinergic			
Convulsions (tonic)					Ganglionic Blockade			
Convulsions (clonic)					Central Blockade			
Piloerection					Antihistaminic			
					Hypertensive			
Depressant					Hypotensive			
Ptosis					Tachycardia			
Sedation					Bradycardia			
Anaesthesia					Diarrhoea			
Ataxia					Emesis			
Loss of righting reflex								
Catatonia								
Analgesia (Tail clip)					Smooth Muscle (g. pig ileum)			
Straub's tail phenomenon					Antiacetylcholine			
Rotating rod test					Antiserotonin			
Loss of placing reflex					Antinicotine			
Loss of pinna reflex					Antihistaminic			
					Anti Barium-Chloride			
Autonomic Effects					Contraction			
Laboured Respiration					Antipyresis (Rats)			
Cyanosis					Diuresis (Rats)			
Blanching					Anti inflammatory test			
Reddening					Carrageenin Oedema (Rats)			
Hypothermia					Cats:			
Abnormal Secretions					Hyperactivity			
Diarrhoea					Restlessness			
Constipation					Decreased activity			
Distress					Nic-Mem relax			
					Vomiting			
					Diarrhoea			
Motor Activity (Mice)					Salivation			
Increased					Aggressiveness			
Decreased					Sleep			
Anti-Convulsant test (Mice)					Motor tone			
Analgesic test					Gait			
b) Chemical					Appetite			
a) Electrical (M.E.S.)					Tremors			
Barbital Sodium Hypnosis					Convulsions			
Anti-reserpine test					Respiration			

Table 2.1b: Prototype observation sheet for cats

PRIMARY SCREENING

Administration Route of Dose:

Solvent:

Date:
Animal: Cat
Sex:
Wt.

	Basal	1 hour	1 hour	1½ hour	2 hours	3 hours	4 hours	24 hours
Convulsion								
Tremors								
Hyperactivity								
Restlessness								
Piloerection								
Decreased activity								
Sleep								
Motor tone								
Gait								
Aggressiveness								
Nictitating membrane								
Pupil dilatation								
Pupil-constriction								
Salivation								
Vomiting								
Urination								
Diarrhoea								
Respiration								
Appetite								

$1/5^{th}$ of approximate LD_{50} dose of a drug obtained via different routes of administration.

The drug effects on central nervous system (CNS) such as depression/stimulation can be evaluated. The most striking effect of depression is decrease in motor activity. In this study, using animals like mice and rats, the drug effects on motor activity can be evaluated using various activity box coupled with electronic gadgets for quantitative measurement of motor activity profiles (e.g. Actophotometer, Jiggle cage).

JIGGLE CAGE:

In this experiment, single animal is placed in a closed cage which is suspending on sensitive spring. The animal's upward and downward movement can be recorded with the help frontal writing lever on a smoked revolving drum. The activity can be recorded preferably at night time (as rodents are nocturnal animals and their activity is more at night time). The activity needs to be recorded for longer time and movements can be measured at different doses so that duration of effect along with dose response relationship can also be determined.

ACTOPHOTOMETER:

In this experiment, motor activity/movements are measured using photocells which are activated when light falling on photocells are cut off by animals crossing the light path. The actophotometer is largely used for evaluating exploratory or forced movements of animals.

In actophotometer, a group of 6 mice are placed and movements are recorded for a fixed interval. Actophotometer records cumulative counts. Thus, effect of a drug on motor activity is recorded at different time intervals following drug treatment. The effect of test drug can be compared with control (vehicle treated) group. Food and water has to be withdrawn 2 hours prior to experiment. The hyperactivity or CNS stimulant as well as CNS depressant activity can be measured using both actophotometer and Jiggle's cage instruments.

Chlorpromazine, reserpine, barbiturates (at low doses), benzodiazepines, hydroxyzine etc can be used as depressants and amphetamine and caffeine can be used as stimulants.

β,β-iminodipropionnitrile (IDPN) when administered to mice induce hyperactivity state (syndrome) which lasts for nearly a month. Mice treated so exhibits continuous circling activity. Chlorpromazine, reserpine and hydroxyzine prevent the agitation and circling of IDPN behaviour in mice and normalize their response to noxious stimulus. Whereas hypnotics like barbiturates completely block the circling behaviour only at hypnotic doses.

MUSCLE RELAXANT ACTIVITY (ROTA-ROD):

The muscle relaxant activity is determined by rota-rod test **(Fig. 2.1)**. In this method, mice weighing (20-25 g) body weight are used. They are trained on a rotating rod (diameter 32 mm, rotating at 12 rpm) and the mice that are able to maintain at least 3 minutes or more on the rod are selected, and randomly divided into different groups (6-8 mice per group). Each group is administered orally vehicle or the test compound and the reference drug. After 30 minutes, mice are placed on the rotating rod at an interval of 30 minutes up to 3 hours. If mice fall down more than once in 3 minutes, test drug effect is considered to be positive, suggesting loss of motor coordination or produce muscle relaxant activity.

Recently, there has been some renewed thinking about the importance of rota-rod method. Instead of just noting "fall off" time, more detailed observations need to be considered that how many times the animal takes to ride. A free ride can be broadly defined as a revolution of the rota-rod during which the animal holds to the rod, rather than walks on it. These free rides are likely to affect the assessment of the drug responses. The performance of mice treated CNS depressant is recorded as either in percentage decrease in performance time on the rotating rod or percentage of animals falling off the rod at a predetermined time. It is observed

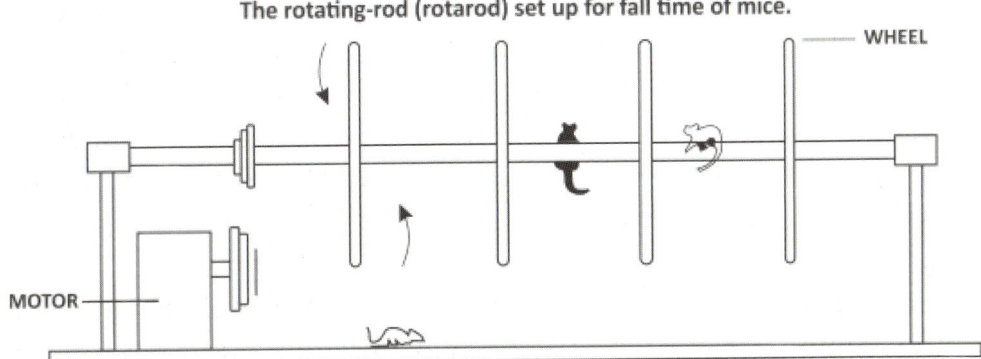

The rotating-rod (rotarod) set up for fall time of mice.

Fig. 2.1: Rota-rod apparatus.

and established that more consistent dose response effect is obtained with Chlorpromazine, diazepam, and for other drugs the dose response effect is observed only when the performance time method of recording is followed.

Plot on a graph paper the percentage mice falling against time intervals to find out the peak drug effect and duration of drug effect. Calculate ED_{50} at peak hour of effect using different doses. Such type of study helps to compare and to determine the potency of different drugs.

AMPHETAMINE AGGREGATION TOXICITY:

Amphetamine administration to mice causes hyperactivity associated with excitement. The hyperactivity is much more pronounced if treated mice are kept in a cage together rather than individually. It is observed that increased stimulation or hyperactivity is almost tenfold at a dose of 14 mg/kg by intraperitoneal route. Such aggregation toxicity is ameliorated or reduced by pre-treatment with major tranquilizers like Chlorpromazine or reserpine. However, minor tranquilizers are found to be ineffective to reduce or prevent the amphetamine aggregation toxicity.

POTENTIATION OF BARBITAL HYPNOSIS (SLEEPING TIME):

In barbital hypnosis test, the most preferred barbiturate is hexobarbital due to its short half life. However, many researchers are using pentobarbital sodium because of its ease of availability and also its fairly short half- life The test needs to be performed at temperature (28-30°C), normal humidity and noise free room. The sleeping time or hypnosis is defined as the time interval between the loss of righting reflex to recovery of the righting reflex of the animal. Generally, sleeping time is prolonged by most of the tranquilizers. Also, a large variety of other substances which are known to affect CNS sensitivity (e.g. Sodium barbital, a non-metabolizing barbiturate) and the drugs known to alter vascular permeability that may affect the entry of barbiturate into the brain. Nevertheless the potentiating effect of barbiturate hypnosis is largely considered as a useful screening method for the evaluation of CNS depressants.

In general, any hyperactivity is associated with drug treatment that impairs the fine balance normally exists in CNS between excitatory and inhibitory stimulus. Hence, CNS stimulation by the drugs resides in adjusting the integration of excitation and inhibitory influences at the level of individual. Thus, it is presumed that any chemical substance produces CNS stimulating activity by one of the following mechanism(s).

a) The enhancement of excitatory neurotransmission
b) Inhibition or antagonism of inhibitory neurotransmission
c) Alter pre-synaptic control of neurotransmitter release.

OPEN FIELD TEST:

The open field is developed originally by Calvin S Hall. The open field test is an experiment used to assay general activity levels and anxiety in rodents in psychoactive drug research. Its dimensions of the apparatus is 50 × 50 × 40 cm and made up of a wooden, open from top and bottom kept on a white table top. The top surface is divided into 25 equal squares i.e. 10 at the centre and 15 at the periphery.

Animals, rats/mice are pre-treated with test drug at different doses one hour prior to the experiment. Diazepam is generally used as a reference drug. During 5 minutes session of the observation, the individual animal is placed at the corner of the apparatus. The exploratory behavioural patterns like ambulation (number of entrance of square with forelimbs), rearing, preening and defecation are recorded. The mean counts of each exploratory parameter (both at the centre and peripheral squares) is computed, analysed and compared with that of the reference drug treatment group.

Some researchers have used Hole-Board test for the evaluation of certain component of behavioural parameters. In such experiments, mouse poking nose into the hole but does not go to the bottom, and is measured quantitatively by the addition of a counting interruption of light beam (electronic device). Alternatively, behavioural parameters are recorded through digital video camera and the video files can be stored in the computer for analysis. (Amos et al, 2003). Behavioral avoidance tests are now well established with the help of the newly designed electronic apparatus with specific behavioural parameters for studying the effect of new compounds on dementia/amnesia.

SCOPOLAMINE-INDUCED AMNESIA:

The test apparatus consists of small chamber connected to a large chamber via guillitone door. In acquisition trials, the animal (rat or mice) is placed in the illuminated compartment at a maximum distance from the guillitone door, and the latency time to enter the dark compartment is measured. After entering the dark compartment, the door is closed automatically and unavoidable foot shock is applied. Animals are randomly divided into different groups (6-8/group). Control group receive either vehicle or normal saline (10 ml/kg by oral route) and test group animals to be administered with the test drug at different doses orally. A dose response curve is plotted or ED_{50} dose (fifty percent effective dose) is calculated for determination of potency of test compound.

The amnesia is produced in animals by administering scopolamine (3 mg/kg i.p.). The animal (mouse/rat) is placed individually 5 minutes after the administration on the bright side of a two-chamber box for training (Vogel, 2002). After brief orientation training session, the mice enter the dark chamber. Once the animal is inside the dark chamber, the door is closed which prevents the mice from escaping, the mice are given electric shock (foot shock-1mA/second) applied through the grid floor. The animal subsequently returns to the home cage. The testing is performed 24 hours later by placing mice again in the bright chamber. The latency in entering the dark chamber within 5 minutes is measured.

Evaluation: The latency to step-through the learning phase and the latency during retention (or resting) test are measured. In this test, a prolongation of the step-through latencies is specific to the experimental situation. An increase of the step-through latency is defined as learning.

In the light-dark model, explorative activity of animal is inhibited by bright illumination, is highly aversive for rodents. However, when placed into a large box connected through a narrow opening with small dark compartment, the animal immediately enters the small dark compartment and spends most of the time there. The time spent in small and large compartments are measured. The animal placed on the brightly lit side of the two-compartment chamber, and the number of crossings between light and dark compartment is used as an auxiliary criteria. Anxiolytics produce a dose dependent increase in crossing.

Caffeine at 3,6,12 and 24 mg/kg doses produce dose dependent increase in locomotion, whereas chlorpromazine at 2,4,8 and 16 mg/kg produce decrease in the locomotion dose dependently.

Motor activity and exploratory time are recorded. The values of the treated group are expressed as percentage of controls. Benzodiazepines and valproate decrease motor activity and increase exploratory time. The anxiolytics produce dose dependent crossing whereas non-anxiolytics do not show such dose dependent response effects.

The advantage of this method is that the relative potency of anxiolytics increase exploratory behaviour in two compartment chamber is totally in agreement with the potency reported in clinical trials. Although the method is time consuming, it is a reliable method for screening anxiolytics.

The computerized automatic systems are available for elevated plus maze and T maze (Technical and Scientific equipment GmBH, D-61348 Hamburg, Germany). Such automatic equipments are helpful to derive more accurate and quantitative results that are useful for an effective assessment of anxiolytics. Latency to enter a mirrored chamber by mice has also been developed for behavioural assay of anxiolytics agents. Toubas et al (1990).

Radial Arm Maze (RAM)

The radial arm maze **(Fig. 2.2)** consists of 8 horizontal arms (57×11) arranged around central platform. The automated doors (20 cm hight) are located at the entrance of each arm. Experimental animals are placed on the platform from which they must collect hidden baits placed in a well at the end of the arms (see **Fig. 2.2**). This type of maze is used to perform short-term memory experimentation in rats. This type of maze can also be used for studying the spatial learning and special memory of animals. (Penley et al 2013, Levin, 1988).

In a standard version of radial arm maze (RAM) test, animals are habituated to the environment placed on the central platform and allowed to explore the maze for a period of 15 minutes per day. Reinforces are scattered on the arms. On habituation (3rd day) the amount of reinforces is reduced to half, and session ends when all 8 arms are visited by the animal. Following habituation, the animals are trained one session per day continuously for 8 days. One piece of reinforce are placed at the end of each arm in a well that hides the food from the sight and animal is allowed to freely explore the maze. Each session continue until
a)   All 8 arms are entered fully
b)   Ten minutes later since the start of the test
c)   Two minutes since the animal's last arm entrance.

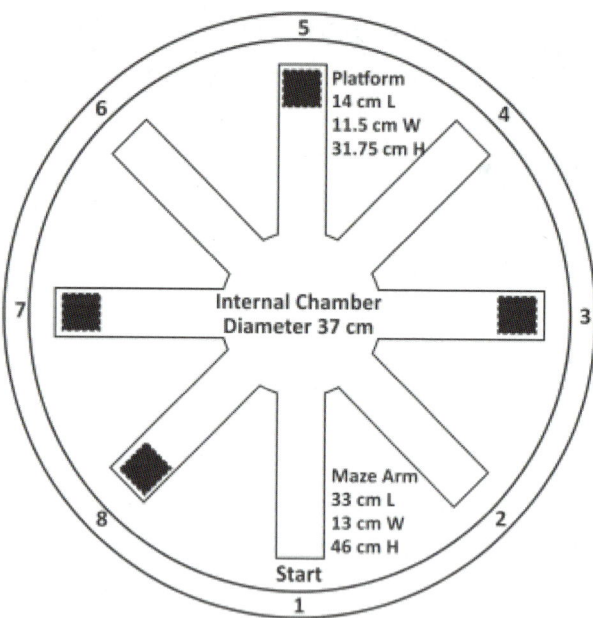

Fig. 2.2: Radial arm maze.

The arm entries are recorded for later analysis. The various other factors such as odour, cues can adversely affect the experimental findings, hence the maze must be thoroughly wiped before placing each and every animal.

a)   The errors in each session (entering the arm that has already been visited is a inherent error [pitfall]) and hence the total number of errors are counted across eight sessions.

b)   The number of precise choices in first 8 arm entries of each session.

c)   The location of the first error in each session.

d)   The number of adjacent arm entries in each session.

e)   The time taken to visit each arms (the total time to complete the session divided by the total number of arm entries).

f)   The number of session to reach the criterion with one error or less averaged error over four consecutive days of training (Tarragon, 2012).

ELEVATED PLUS MAZE:

This test has been widely used and periodically validated to evaluate anxiety component in rodents. The apparatus is fabricated using Plexiglass and has two open arms (30 cm × 5 cm) and two closed arm (30 cm × 5 cm) walls. The open and closed arms are connected by central platform (50 cm × 5 cm). The maze has four-foot stand platform having a height of elevation of 38.5 cm from the floor **(Fig. 2.3)**. The platform and the lateral walls of the closed arm are made of black

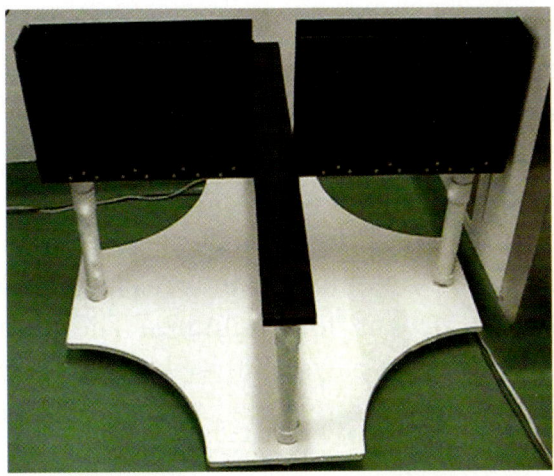

Fig. 2.3: Elevated Plus Maze

acrylic. Rats or mice of either sex are used. They are randomly divided into various groups (6/group) as per design or objectives of the experiment. Each animal is placed at the centre of the maze, facing one of the enclosed arms. The number of entries and time spent by the animal during 5 minutes test period is measured. The complete entry can be considered only if the animal is placing all the four paws in the arm. The test needs to be repeated to ensure reliability of the experimental findings. The effect profile of a drug such as peak effect, duration and dose response effect are determined. (Walf et al, 2007) (Braun et al 2011).

Y-MAZE TEST:

The Y-maze is widely used behavioural task in neuroscience for studying spatial learning and memory.

Y-shaped maze with three white opaque plastic arms at a 120° angle from each other. This test is devised to study the effect of drugs on spontaneous motor activity

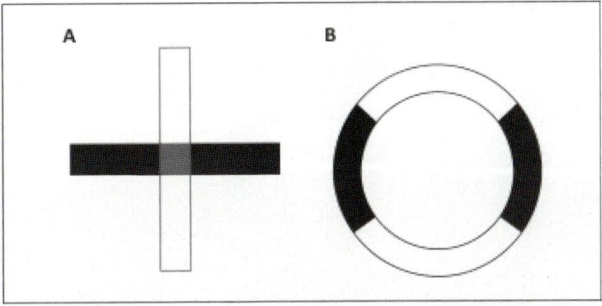

Fig. 2.4: (A) Elevated plus maze. (B) Elevated zero mazes. Black indicates enclosed areas, white indicates open areas, and gray represents centre region in the Plus maze.

as well as motor co-ordination status. It is also used for the learning task, such as special reference memory task in which the animal has to learn which of the arms is baited with a food reward. Furthermore, the method is also used to discriminate between the effects of exercise on memory acquisition, and long-term memory retention. This test can also be extended to quantify cognitive deficits in transgenic strains of mice, and routinely used for evaluating new chemical entities for their effect on cognition. Generally, mice are used and are placed in a symmetrical shaped runway (33 cm × 38 cm × 13 cm) for 3 minutes. The numbers of the entrance into the maze with four feet (four paws onto each arm) are counted. The number of entries and number of traits are recorded to calculate percentage alterations **(Fig. 2.5)**.

In the Y-maze study, the paradigms used are, mice had to learn which of the two arms forming the Y is baited with the food. A day prior to the start of the training, mice are allowed to freely explore the maze for 5 minutes. Subsequently, they received two trials, one in which the food is kept in the left arm and the second one in which the food is positioned in the right arm. During the training procedure, only one of the two arms contained a food crumb. For half of the mice this is in the left arm, and for the other half this is in the right arm. In order to avoid any stress related artefact, during the learning process, mice are not handled by the experimenter but are allowed to voluntarily enter the maze. Whenever a mouse visited one of the two arms, the trapdoor of the non-visited arm is generally closed. The mouse is allowed to eat the small piece of food, and there after the mouse re-enters its home cage, the arm connected to the home cage is closed. After thorough cleaning of the arms, the mouse is allowed to enter the maze again for the next trial.

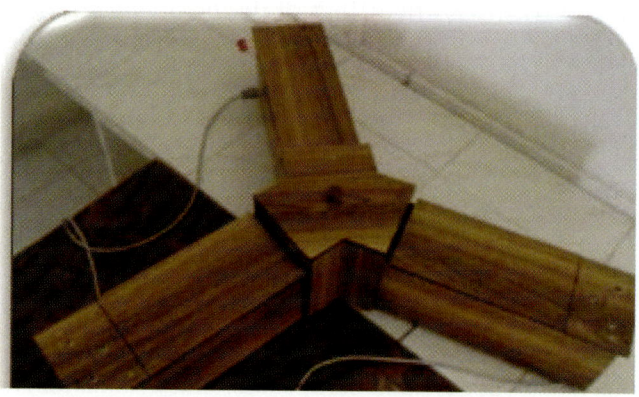

Fig. 2.5: Y maze apparatus.

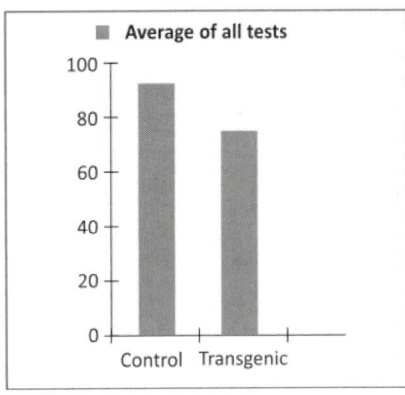 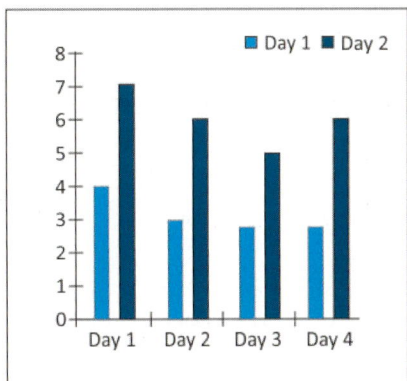

Fig 2.5a: (A) Y maze Spontaneous Alteration Activity (B) Y maze number of entries

This test is particularly useful in measuring cognitive deficits in transgenic animals assessing hippocampal (learning area) damage and correlating the effects of drug to cognition related aspects (Ishwar Tony et al, 2013, Shoji et al, 2012).

CONDITIONED AVOIDANCE RESPONSE:

The effect of drugs on conditioned responses in experimental animals has been used as a screening procedure for major tranquilizers (Cook and Weidley, 1957). A pole climbing apparatus **(Fig. 2.6)** consists of a base with an electrified grid and a buzzer arrangement. The pole attached to the lid which can be removed after the rat has climbed onto the pole. A group of rats are trained in the apparatus. During training the buzzer and shock are simultaneously applied. This differs from the classical conditioning methods where the unconditioned stimulus (electric shock) follows the conditioned stimulus (buzzer) after a very brief interval.

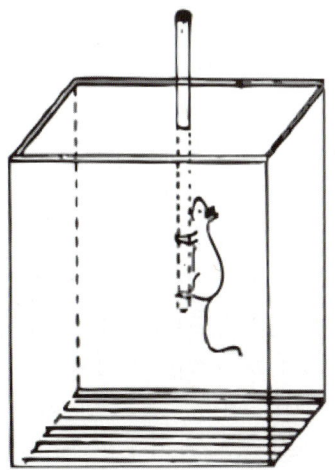

Fig. 2.6: Pole climbing apparatus.

The shock (80 volts, 5 pulses/second) is applied through a stimulator to the floor grid. The rats are shocked intermittently for varying lengths of time, each time the shock lasting not more than 30 seconds. The rats are trained initially 3 times a day. After one week's training, only the buzzer is tried and the shock is applied only when the rats do not climb the pole with the buzzer.

The rats usually learn to climb the pole within 3 seconds of the buzzer in about 2 weeks training. Reinforcement runs have to be repeated 2 or 3 times a week.

The trained rats are selected and randomly divided into various groups (6-8 rats/group) and test drugs are administered in various doses, and dose response effect to buzzer is recorded at 15,30,60,120 min. Non treated group is considered as control, and a positive control group is treated with reference drug for comparison. The conditioned stimulus when applied is completely blocked if the rat does not climb within 30 seconds. Shock is applied to find out the presence of unconditioned response (UR). Blocking UR (shock) response is considered as an indication either of motor paralysis or severe toxic effects. A dose response relationship in a time recovery curve should be plotted. Conditioned response is blocked effectively by most of the major tranquilizers.

MAO INHIBITION TEST :

Hydrazine and non-hydrazine anti-depressants show an intensity of MAO inhibition which parallels to an extent of their clinical relevance as anti-depressant drugs. This concept led to the introduction of MAO inhibition as a parameter to study the potency of anti-depressant drugs. Reserpine and tetrabenazine induce CNS depression, ptosis, miosis and fall in body temperature, potentiation of hexobarbital sleeping time and blocking of conditioned response. These agents also reduce 5-HT and NE content in the brain. These effects are blocked or reversed by iproniazid and other MAO inhibitors. MAO inhibitors are known only to prevent the early reserpine effects, but cannot reverse the total effects once they are fully established. In mice and rats, imipramine and amitriptyline reverse the effects of small doses of tetrabenazine or reserpine. The reversal of reserpine-induced hypothermia has also been used as a screening parameter to evaluate antidepressant activity in rabbits and rats. Also refer Evaluation methods of drug activities described in pharmacometrics (Vogel).

BEHAVIOURAL DESPAIR IN RATS, A NEW MODEL RESPONDS TO ANTI-DEPRESSANTS:

Rats when forced to swim in a cylinder from which they cannot escape, rats after an initial struggle of vigorous attempts try to adopt a characteristic immobile posture/immobility which can be easily and glaringly identifiable. Such immobility is reduced by various clinically used anti-depressant agents at certain dose level, which is similar to reduced spontaneous motor activity observed in an open field test. Anti-depressant thus distinguished from psycho-stimulants, which decreases immobility, whereas psychoactive major tranquilizers known to enhance the same. Immobility is also reduced by electro convulsion shock. Rapid eye movement (REM), sleep deprivation and "enhancement" has also been reported. In this experiment, the findings largely suggest that immobility represents a state of reduced mood in the rat that seems to be sensitive to anti-depressant drugs. Certain positive experimental findings with atypical anti-depressants, imprindole and mianserin point out that this model represents endogenous depression model and is useful for screening new class of anti-depressants.

In some other type of experiment, rats are placed in glass or plastic rectangular tank (height 30 cm, breadth 30 cm and depth 15-20 cm) filled with water. Two type of swimming tests are conducted. The initial 15 minutes pre-test period should be performed and 24 hour later followed by 6-minute test period. Initial experiments are conducted to train rats for acclimatization. In actual experiments, each animal is administered with the test drug doses and then placed in water tank for 6 minutes and behavioural parameters are recorded, during the last 4 minutes.
1) Immobility: Floating in water being motionless.
2) Swimming with its full movements of limbs.
3) Animal trying active movements mainly by fore-paws on the wall of tank.

Using proper scoring system for each behavioural parameter mentioned above, the drug effects can be studied and evaluated. A dose response curve can be plotted and potency can be assessed by comparing with the standard anti-depressant drug. (Paulo et al, 2005) .

THE TAIL SUSPENSION TEST :

It is a mouse behavioural test useful in the screening of anti-depressant drug, and also useful in assessing of other manipulations that are known to influence the depression related behaviours. A mouse is suspended by the tail with an adhesive tape from the lever, in such a position that cannot escape or hold on to nearby surface. In this experiment, typically 6 minutes duration, the resulting escape oriented behaviours are quantified and recorded. The total duration of the test (6 minutes) can be divided into periods of agitation and immobility. The tail suspension test is designed as an alternate choice for the forced swimming test. However, the basic principle of both the models remains same. The mice suspended by their tails, intrinsically endeavour to get away, from the adverse circumstances. As a result of the fizzled endeavour to get away, the mice experience despair and become immobile. The extent and degree of immobility is considered to be associated with depressive like condition of the mice, and is significantly diminished by the clinically used anti-depressant drugs. Many psychotropic drugs, amphetamine,amitryptline, atropine, disimpramine, mianserine, nomifensive and violoxazine, and other anti-depressant drugs decrease the duration of immobility as do psychostimulants and atropine.

If coupled with the measurement of locomotor activity in different conditions, the test can help to differentiate between the locomotor stimulant doses and anti-depressant doses. Diazepam treatment show significant increase in the duration of immobility time period.

Experimental procedure: In the tail suspension test (TST) the mice are suspended by their tails on a suspension bar or table using adhesive tape, and the height should be kept 50 cm over the floor. The tape ought to be connected to the ending part of the tail of the mouse with 2-3 mm of the tail staying outside the tape.

When the tape has been appended to the mouse tail, affix the middle part of the tape to the suspension bar.

Start the video recording device connected to the computer when scoring is carried out.

Once the experiment time has elapsed (6 minutes), the mouse is kept back in the home cage.

Analysis: The duration of tail suspension test is 6 minutes. It is slightly different than other followed anti-depressant method, such as forced swimming test. The entire session is scored. This is largely due to the fact that animals show immobility earlier in the TST.

The prime scoring parameter is the immobility time. The other essential part of TST investigation is the uniform recognition of movements that are scored as true mobility. Initially animals show distinctly escaping behaviour-like arriving at the suspension bar, rigorous shaking of the body and movements of the appendages (akin to running). All such behavioural patterns certainly constitute mobility. After some time, such behaviour dies down and gets to be subtle and immobility status.

Interpretation: Like forced swimming test, in this experiment, the animals are set in a preventable yet maintained modestly distressing circumstances. Escape behaviour absence is considered as immobility. TST is a test approved for assessment of anti-depressant like medications; additionally it is useful to assess the impacts of ecological, neurobiological and hereditary controls (Cryonet al, 2005).

ACUTE RESTRAINT STRESS (ARS):

Mice are immobilised for a period of 7 hours using individual rodent restraint device made of Plexiglass fenestrate, restraining all physical movement without causing pain because pain involvement in any type of movements is ethically not permitted. Anti-depressant drug fluoxetine (20 mg/kg p.o.) is administered 1 hour prior to ARS and then animals are subjected to ARS using above mentioned device. Pretreatment of fluoxetine reduce significantly the immobility time. The ARS stress is frequently used to induce depressive behaviour in experimental animals. Animals are immobilized for longer periods exhibit unavoidable physical and mental stress which is difficult to adapt and finally lead to increase in immobility time in ARS test or in forced swimming test.

THE OLFACTORY BULBECTOMIZED RAT AS A MODEL FOR DEPRESSION:

The olfactory bulb removal in rodents results in the disruption of hippocampal neurogenesis, akin to the mechanism implicated in depression. Olfactory bulb extends to various brain region mainly hippocampus, cerebral cortex and amygdale etc and ablation of bulbs leads to behavioural, neurochemical, neuroendo-crinological and neuroimmune changes that is akin to the changes seen in depressed patients.

The major behavioural changes observed after olfactory bulbectomized in animals are enhanced nocturnal hyperactivity in a 24 hr home cage activity open field type, deficit in memory mainly reflected by passive avoidance behaviour, also in the Morris water maze, and 8 arm radial maze, increased open arm entries in the elevated plus maze and changes in food by motivated and conditioned taste aversion behaviour.

The neurochemical changes such as nor-adrenergic, serotonergic, cholinergic, gamma-aminobutyric acid (GABA) and glutamic acid are also associated with the olfactorybulbectomized animals. The other changes are: reduced neutrophil phagocytosis, lymphocyte mitogenesis, lymphocyte number and negative acute/phase proteins. It appears that olfactory bulb removal causes a major dysfunction of the cortical – hippocampal-amygdala circuit that underlies behavioural and other changes. The most commonly observed behavioural indicators of the anti-depressant activity are attenuation of the olfactory bulbectomized related hyperactivity in the open field. The other behavioural, neurotransmitters and immune changes associated with depression are attenuated only by chronic anti-depressant drug treatment.

Tricyclic–anti-depressants, (amitriptyline, despiramine), atypical agents (mianserine), selective serotonin reuptake inhibitors (paroxetine, sertraline, fluvoxamine) reversible inhibitors of monoamine oxidase A (moclobemide) as well as putative anti-depressants such as 5-hydroxytryptamine 1A ($5HT_{1A}$) agonist (zalospirone, ipsapirone), non-competitive N-methyl-D-aspartate antagonist (MK-801) and alprazolam, adinazolam exhibit anti-depressant-like activity in this model. Hence, this model is considered to be qualitatively similar to many aspects of behavioural symptoms observed in depressive patients.

Recently, neuroimmune mechanisms are considered as a central to the development of depressive symptoms, and emerging evidence is beginning to identify the neural circuits involved in cytokine-induced depressive disorders. The rodent experimental models of inflammation related depression can be divided into different groups (a) depression induced by exposure to inflammation related agents and (b) by genetic manipulations of inflammation related genes.

Systemic lipopolysaccharide challenge in rodent increases inflammatory reaction in the central nervous system and associated with behaviours such as reduced motor activity, reduced food and water intake, and enhanced sleep, serial and social withdrawals, which resemble to depressive symptoms in humans. Polyinosinic acid-polycytidylic acid has also been used instead of lipopolysaccharide to induce maternal immune activation in animal model, which increases depression-like behaviours in the offspring of inflicted dams.

There are specific soluble cytokine receptors on blood brain barrier, by binding to such proinflammatory cytokines can activate neurons and recruit local microglia to initiate and maintain sickness behavior. This suggest immune-related mechanisms with depression. Furthermore, proinflammatory cytokines also stimulate the hypothalamus-pituitary-adrenal axis (HPA) thereby helping to affective pathogenesis of depression.

Many other models used are: social defeat model in which defeat rodent shows a number of physiological changes such as reduced sexual behavior, increased defensive behavior, enhanced anxiety, decreased motor activity and exploratory activity, changes in circadian rhythmicity, decreased food intake and body weight, sleep disturbances and impaired immune functions. Even HPA axis is activated, which are similar to symptoms of depression in humans including many experimental models of depression.

REMOVAL OF OLFACTORY BULB, SURGICAL PROCEDURE :

Rats are anaesthetized with vetbutal (65 mg/kg i.p.) and removal of bilateral olfactory bulb is performed. Following exposure of the skull 2 mm diameter holes are drilled at the points 7 mm anterior to bregma and 2 mm either side of the midline. Then olfactory bulbs (OB) are removed by suction and holes are tilted with haemostatic sponge to stop the bleeding and the skin is closed. Sham operated animals are treated the same way but the bulbs are left intact. After surgery, the animals are kept in cage (4 animals/cage). Animals are given 14 days to recover following surgery. Animals are handled carefully to avoid aggressiveness. The drug treatment can be initiated after 2-3 weeks of surgery. The open field test and the passive avoidance test are performed after the test drug treatment (both acute and chronic). The test procedure of open field and passive avoidance are already mentioned earlier in this chapter. The effect of drug on olfactory bulbectomized (OB) induced behavioural abnormality such as hyperactivity in the open field test as well as deficit in step down passive avoidance can also be studied.

Neurochemical changes such as OB-induced low levels of 5-HT, noradrenaline, high 5-Hydroxyindoleacetic acid (5HIAA), 4-Hydroxyphenylacetic acid (DOPAC) in hippocampus are observed. Anti-depressant drugs treatment completely reverse such neurotransmitters alterations in OB rats.

The other behavioural alterations observed in OB are hyperactivity in a brightly illuminated open field, and in a novel cage as well as in T-maze. Further OB also exhibit increased exploratory behaviour in the novel object test and the T-maze test. Most of the animal models described above have demonstrated that treatment with antidepressant drugs improves behavioural alterations significantly in all the above mentioned models.

CHRONIC MILD STRESS INDUCED ANHEDONIA- A RELIABLE ANIMAL MODEL OF DEPRESSION:

Chronic sequential exposure of a variety of mild and unpredictable stressors (21 days) (food-water deprivation, temperature alterations) causes a decrease in responsiveness to rewards in rats. Such chronic exposure to stressful conditional also induce long lasting changes of behavioral, neuro-immune and neuro-endocrinological variables-changes resembling reward functions like anhedonia (increased threshold for intra-cranial self-administration) and are reversed by acute/chronic administration of anti-depressant drugs. This model provides better insight into the neurobiology and pathophysiology of depression.

Some traditional anti-depressant animal models such as reserpine reversal, amphetamine potentiation are not used regularly due to poor correlation of experimental findings and less reliability. The most valid and acceptable models are: intracranial self-administration, chronic stress and learned helplessness in rats and primate separation model. The chronic mild stress and learned helplessness test in rat model show that depression like behaviour is accompanied by periphery and central inflammation, neuronal cell damage, impaired neurogenesis and apoptosis in the hippocampus. Alterations in sleep architecture and disturbances in circadian rhythms are observed in electroencephalogram (EEG). The various biochemical changes associated are: increased interleukin-1β, tumour necrosis factor-α, IL-6, nuclear factor $\kappa\beta$, cyclo-oxygenase-2, expression of toll-like receptors and lipid peroxidation. Anti-neurogenic effects reducs brain derived neurotropic factor (BDNF) levels, and apoptosis with reduced levels of BCl-2 (B-cell lymphoma- 2) and BAG1 (BCl-2 associated anthogen 1) and increased levels of capase-3. Anti-depressants decrease central and peripheral IL-1β,TNF-α and IL-6 levels and stimulate neuronal differentiation, synaptic effects on the expression of different neurotropic factors such as trkB (Tropomyosin related kinase B), the receptor for BDNF and attenuate apoptotic pathways by stimulating BCl-2 and BCl-xl proteins and suppressing capase-3.

The learned helplessness test (LHT) in rat is one of the well validated animal models. The significance is that repeated exposure to uncontrollable and stressful events in life causes people to feel that they are losing control which sometime manifest depressive like behaviors. In this, animal are exposed one day or over several days to unavoidable and uncontrollable shocks (e.g. Tail-shock, foot-shock in shuttle boxes) in which animals develop deficits in escape, cognitive and rewarded behaviors. The helpless behaviour is assessed by carefully analysing the performance in an active escape test in terms of latency to press a lever or cross the closed doors (described in earlier tests).

In this test, excellent face and predictive validity make LHT model interesting for exploration of pathophysiology of depression. Since it requires high intensity stressors to induce behavioural alterations, which often raises ethical problems and most of the symptoms do not last long enough, following cessation of the uncontrollable shock.

However, chronic mild stress does induce most reliable model of depression. Further, the model results in long lasting changes of behavioral, neuro-immune and neuro-endocrinological variable and pathological changes resembling reward function including decreased intra-cranial self-stimulation, reflecting anhedonia which are reversed by chronic anti-depressant treatment.

There are many models such as social defeat stress (SDStr) which is a chronic recurring factor in the lives of all higher animal species. Since majority of stress stimuli in humans lead to physiological changes that are of social nature, the SDStr is also gaining increasing attention as it has good predictive validity. In this model only male rodents are used. The maternal deprivation model is the most widely used early life stress model. The maternal separation results in increased anxiety and depression like behaviour and increased HPA (Hypothalamic-pituitary-adrenal axis) response in adulthood.

Olfactory Bulbectomy surgical procedure	Recovery period Day 1- Day 14	Treatment schedule Day 15 - Day 28	Behavioural Analysis (Open field and Forced Swimming test) Day 29 and 30th

Fig. 2.7: Evaluation Studies.

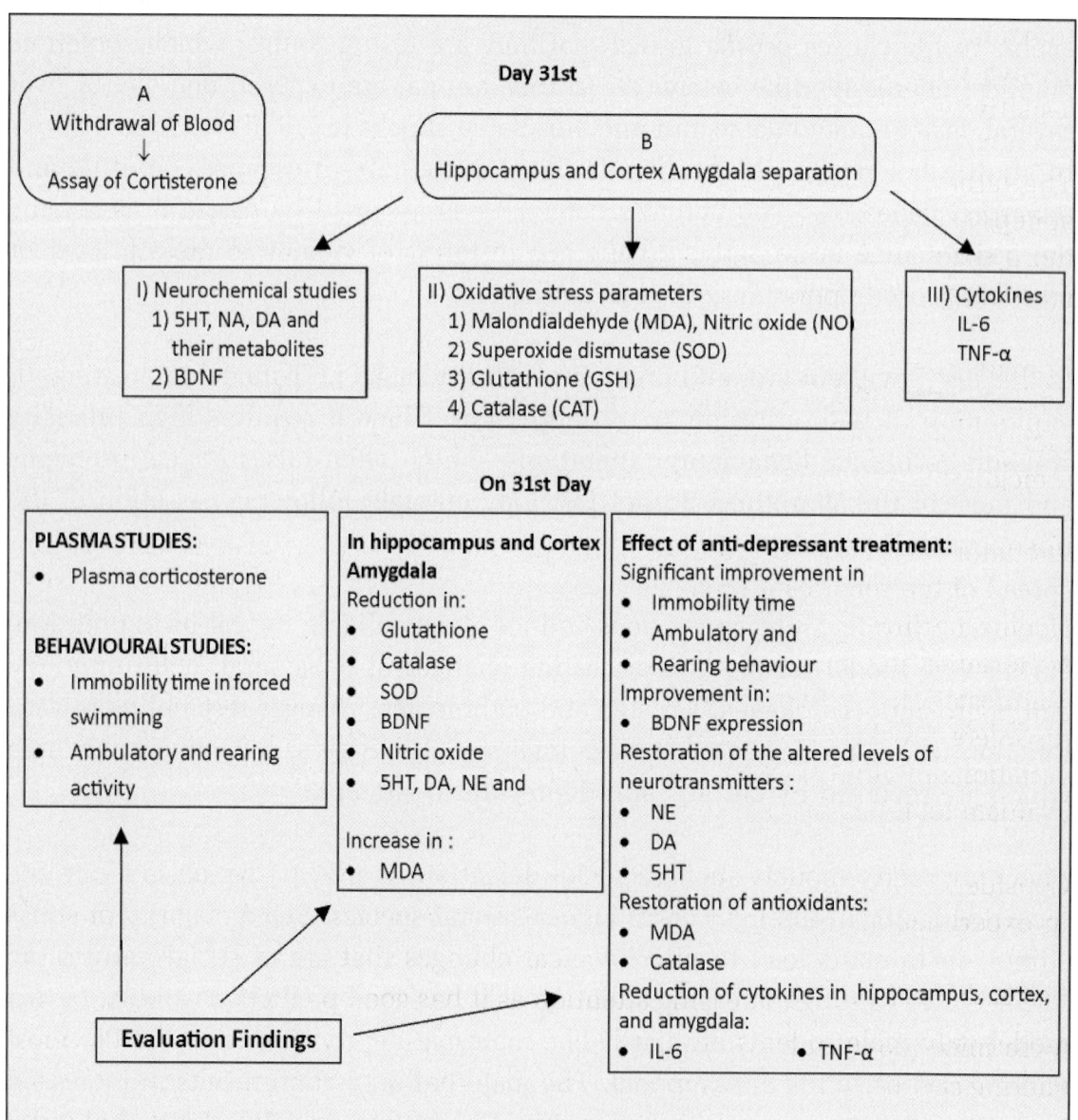

Fig. 2.8: Evaluation findings

ANTI-CONVULSANT DRUG SCREENING:

Drugs that are intended for the treatment of epilepsy/convulsive disorders in man are called anti-convulsants or anti-epileptic drugs. The etiology of convulsions is numerous. Most of the animal models or techniques used for screening anti-convulsant drugs are aimed at evaluating epileptic activity. Human epilepsy is not a single disease, but a syndrome with variety of manifestations. Epilepsy (derived from a Greek word for seizures) is not a single phenomenon but a group of chronic seizure disorders having heterogeneous and a common sudden and transient seizures, loss or brief disturbance of consciousness usually, but not always with characteristic convulsions, and at times with autonomic hyper-sensitivity.

The father of modern concepts of epilepsy, John Hughling Jakson postulated epilepsy as occasional, sudden, excessive, rapid and local discharges of gray matter more than 100 years ago. The same has been confirmed by modern electro-physiology techniques.

Convulsions are correlated with abnormal and excessive discharge in the brain which are normally recorded on electroencephalogram (EEG), neuro-imaging techniques such as magnetic resonance imaging (MRI), positron emission tomography (PET) which are capable of identifying abnormalities in patients.

Excitatory neurotransmitters are thought to be involved in the beginning and spread of the seizures discharge, and the inhibitory neurotransmitters viz GABA, glycine, taurine and ionic conductance modifications are believed to be responsible for termination of seizure activity. However, the findings of these techniques and manifestations of functional hyperactivity differs in different types of epileptic disorders. Difference in such factors is sometimes accompanied by considerable variations in clinical drug response. Therefore, a battery of tests are necessary to evaluate total profile of the test drug in the laboratory.

Considering such pathological features, the different types of seizures are simulated in experimental animals for evaluation of anti-convulsant drugs.

SUPRAMAXIMAL ELECTRIC SHOCK:

Male mice (25-30 g body weight) are selected and brief electric shock (150 mA altering current, 0.2 sec) is applied through corneal electrodes that cause seizures-tonic flexon-tonic extension of roughly 10 sec followed by clonic jerks and sometimes death (due to post tonic asphyxias).

The drugs (e.g. diphenylhydantoin) which are clinically effective in grandmal seizures abolish tonic extension without causing neurological impairment and this is the basic principle of standard screening test for evaluating drug against grandmal.

Dose response relationship for standard test drugs are determined by giving groups of animals 4 or more various doses of the drug, and subjecting them to maximal electric shock (MES) at the peak activity time of the drug.

The duration of anti-convulsants effect is determined by a time response graph from the data of MES test at various time intervals following drug treatment.

Epileptic seizures are broadly classified into partial and generalized seizures **(Table 2.3)**. Partial seizures can be correlated with the damage to the brain, whereas generalized seizures manifest without any definite cause.

Table 2.3: Classification of Seizures

Type of seizures	Subtypes
Partial seizures	• Simple partial seizures • Complex partial seizures • Partial seizures, secondary generalized Seizures
Convulsive or Non-convulsive generalized seizures	• Petitmal • Tonic-clonic convulsions • Clonic-myoclonic seizures • Infantile spasms

Among these types, grandmal epilepsy is the most common and is partially associated with the spasm of all muscles and unconsciousness. The petit mal epilepsy (absence of seizures) is largely prevalent in children in which there is no loss of consciousness and tonic spasm of muscle. Status epilepticus is the state of continuous tonic-clonic convulsions without intermission.

Chemical agents used in inducing convulsions in animal:

Administration of pentenyltetrazol (55-65 mg/kg i.p.), a cerebral stimulant to mice or rats induce clonic convulsions (whole body shake) and at higher doses produce tonic convulsions.

The clonic convulsions in different animal models can be prevented by drugs that are clinically effective in petit mal.

Many other electro-convulsants which intervene in GABA synthesis and/or receptors or intervention of glycine receptors in spinal cord produce convulsions. Strychnine (spinal cord stimulant and glycine receptor blockers) produces continuous convulsions of both clonic and tonic nature which are enhanced in the presence of stressful agents.

Picrotoxin (a GABA-receptor blocker) alters functions of chloride channels at 3.5 mg/kg s.c and isonicotonic acid hydrazide (INH), (GAD inhibitor reduce GABA synthesis that results in its inhibition) and 6-mercapto-propionic acid (a GABA inhibitor) produce initially clonic convulsions followed by tonic convulsions. Four amino-pyridine (13.3 mg/kg, s.c), a non-NMDA type of excitatory amino acid receptor blocker also induces convulsions.

Chronic-focal seizures are produced by applying alumina cream to the motor cortex of the monkey or other species, which eventually lead to spontaneous convulsions that generalize from the focal onset. This causes reduction of number of terminal and small neurons that contain glutamate decarboxylase are decreased within this focii and adjacent tissue. This event inhibits the functions of inhibitory pathways that utilize GABA as congruent with the production of epilepti form firing (discharges) in a group of neurons exposed to drugs that affects the function of GABA, including picrotoxin, pentenyltetrazol and bicucline and penicillin.

Evaluation: Test animals are tested a day before and after the test drugs are treated and compared with the untreated control group. The critical parameters are onset of convulsions, duration of convulsions, and status of animal after 30 minutes and 24 hours including percentage of mortality.

The other model used is an inbred strain of Mongolian gerbil in which slowly develop (55 days) after birth myoclonic, tonic or clonic seizures. The most striking observation (microscopically) in the animal model is an increase of number of neurons and terminals that contain GABA especially in hippocampus region. However, the terminals appear to be located in inhibitory basket cells eventually paving way to the notion of epileptogenesis by non-inhibition.

Chronic focal seizures is also produced in rats by administration of subconvulsive dose of pentenyltetrazol or by electrically stimulating (8 mA current 60 Hz for 4 seconds) daily in discrete areas (right amygdale) of brain in animals (such as rats/mice) produce seizures. This is considered as animal is kindled out and described as kindling epilepsy. Such type of seizures closely resembles to chronic epilepsy. Many clinically used anti-epileptic drugs inhibit such type of epilepsy. A dose related anti-epileptic activity can be studied and compared with standard anti-epileptic drugs.

Clinically used anti-epileptic drug: Diphenyl hydantoin, Phenobarbital, sodium valproate, carbamazepine, primidone, ethosuximide, trimethadone, benzodiazepines, gabapentin, lamotrigine, vigabatrin, felbamate, topiramate.

ANTI-PARKINSON DRUG SCREENING METHODS:

The disease was first described by physician James Parkinson in 1817 and described it as the shaking Palsy. The etiopathology of this disease is not understood to a great extent. With the explanation of Prof Tretiakoff, that in parkinsonism there is great a amount of loss of neurons in substantia nigra pars compacta of mid brain. Subsequently, the role of dopamine and its depletion from basal ganglia is found to be the major causative factor for parkinsonism.

This is followed by in depth studies of pathophysiology, neuropharmacology and neurochemistry of parkinsonism for better understanding of the genesis of disease process. It was observed that it is a chronic passive degenerative disorder of extra pyramidal system in central nervous system, and largely due to imbalance between dopamine and cholinergic neurons. The major clinical symptoms associated with parkinsonism are: rigidity, akinesia, fine tremors at rest, decreased movements, anxiety, depression and sleep disturbances. The autonomic symptoms are excessive salivation, mask like facial expression, typical defective posture, hunched back, excessive blinking, decreased speech volume and loss of cognition as the disease progress.

Various agents are used as a tool to produce animal models of Parkinsonism. 1, 2, 3, 6-methyl-phenyl-tetrahydropyridine (MPTP), a product formed during pethidine manufacturing and produces symptoms akin to parkinsonism. Tremorine, oxotremorine (muscarinic antagonists), reserpine induced circling behaviour in neostraital lesioned rats are also used to simulate Parkinson's disease.

Injection of 6-hydroxydopamine (6OHDM) 8 μg into the anterior zona compacta of the substantia nigra using stereotaxic apparatus following atlas of Konig and Klippel. Ipsilateral or contralateral to the lesion are recorded on an automatic printout counter for every 15 minutes intervals for a period of 1-2 hours. Each rat is injected d-amphetamine 2.5 mg/kg i.p. for ipsilateral circling and placed immediately in a circling chamber for 2 hours. For contralateral circling apomorphine 1 mg/kg is used and recorded circling for 1 hour.

Animal Models used in Anti-Parkinson drug screening:

The Zebrafish (*Danio rarivo*) has been used in neurotoxicity studies including genetic model, developmental biology, and motor neuron diseases. As some regions of its CNS, such as the hypothalamus, optic tracts of olfactory system, spinal cord and cranial nerves including striatal, show a clear structural homology to the relevant areas of the human brain. Furthermore, mammalian neuro-transmitter system such as GABA, glutamate, dopamine, norepinephrine, 5HT, histamine, ACh are also present in zebrafish although difference in expression pattern is observed. The experimental procedure involves selection of adult male or female Zebrafish from a reliable breeder. Fishes are maintained on special food 3 times/day, 10-14 light-dark cycle in a rectangular tank (LXWXH; 25 cm $\times$ 16.5 cm $\times$ 12.5 cm) filled with aerated water at temperature (25$\pm$1°C).

Toxins like paraquat, rotenone and others are used. Prior to actual experiment, pilot experiments are performed to find out appropriate concentration of rotenone at which the explorative motility of Zebrafish is affected, but not causing mortality. The concentration of rotenone 5.0-5.5 mg/L is used and treated for 21 days, that elicited significant reduction in motility and survived up to 4 weeks. The test drugs are administered at different doses by intramuscular route using Hamilton syringe for 21 days daily along with toxin (rotenone). Control group fish received vehicle or normal saline by same route for asimilar period.

Evaluation of motor activity:

The evaluation of motor activity is performed by drawing 3 vertical lines on the tank at equidistance and dividing the tank area into 4 zones (the length of each zone is 6.25 cm). The locomotor activity is measured by counting the number of lines that zebra fish crosses. This helps to calculate total distance travelled by the fish in a unit time interval and the activity is expressed in terms of number of cross lines/5 minutes.

Rotenone (toxin) produce decrease in motor activity and drug preventing neurodegeneration improves motility. For example, Curcumin, L-Dopa, ellagic acid and others have been demonstrated to improve the motility of Zebrafish: *Dmelanogaster* has been used as an alternative animal method for screening drugs/compounds in neurodegenerative diseases like PD, Alzheimer's disease and others.

Experimental Procedure:

Dmelanogaster wild type, Cantor special strain is used. The flies are grown in a glass vial (2.5 cm × 6.5 cm) filled with growing media (8.3% w/v maize flour; 5% w/v glucose, 2.5% w/v sucrose; 1.5% w/v agar; 2% w/v Brewer yeast powder, 0.04% w/v propionic acid; 0.6% w/v orthophosphoric acid; 0.7% w/v methyl hydrobenzoate) at 23°C and 55% relative humidity and keeping 12 h dark/light cycle. Male (8 days old) adult flies are selected and divided into various groups (6-8 each/group).

Negative control (untreated), positive control group flies are exposed to rotenone 500μg, and test group flies are exposed rotenone 500μg + test drug (ellagic acid). The total food medium contained volume of 1% DMSO$_4$, rotenone, rotenone+ test drug. The flies are exposed to various treatment mentioned above for 7 days. While carrying out experiment, flies are maintained at 23°C. The motor activity is evaluated using negative geotaxis assay and experiments are performed during light-cycle only. Flies are transferred into graduated flat bottom glass tube (length 25 cm × 2 cm diameter) and allowed to adapt for a brief period (5-7 minutes). The tube is gently tapped (as stimulus) at the bottom and observed for the climbing activity (a total of 20 flies used in 3 groups). Motor activity is expressed as percent flies climbing a minimum distance of 10 cm in one minute. Rotenone exposed flies don't climb the glass tube. The test drug treatment may improve the motility of flies. Using this procedure, the percent protection of by the test drug can be calculated which represents the improvement or prevention of neurodegeneration. In such experiments, one can demonstrate improvement in locomotor performance, and consequently the drug effect on the neurodegeneration process is also assessed.

References:

1. Amos, S., Binda, L., Akah, P., Wambebe, C., & Gamaniel, K. (2003). Central inhibitory activity of the aqueous extract of Crinum giganteum. Fitoterapia, 74(1-2), 23-28.

2. Chourbaji, S., Zacher, C., Sanchis-Segura, C., Dormann, C., Vollmayr, B., & Gass, P. (2005). Learned helplessness: validity and reliability of depressive-like states in mice. Brain research protocols, 16(1-3), 70-78.

3. Cook, L., & Weidley, E. (1957). Behavioral effects of some psychopharmacological agents. Annals of the New York Academy of Sciences, 66(1), 740-752.

4. Cryan, J.F., Mombereau, C., & Vassout, A. (2005). The tail suspension test as a model for assessing antidepressant activity: review of pharmacological and genetic studies in mice. Neuroscience & Biobehavioral Reviews, 29(4-5), 571-625.

5. Dohare, P., Garg, P., Jain, V., Nath, C., & Ray, M. (2008). Dose dependence and therapeutic window for the neuroprotective effects of curcumin in thromboembolic model of rat. Behavioural brain research, 193(2), 289-297. D

6. D Ishwar Tony et al, Evaluation of Memory Enhancement Activity and Shock Motivated Brightness Discrimination Response by using Y-Maze, Research Journal of Pharmaceutical, Biological and Chemical Sciences; 4(2013); 136-142.

7. Dorr, M., Steinberg, H., Tomkiewicz, M., Joyce, D., Porsolt, R. D., & Summerfield, A. (1971). Persistence of dose related behaviour in mice. Nature, 231(5298), 121.

8. HG Vogel, WH Vogel, Drug Discovery and Evaluation: Pharmacological Assays,Springer- 3rd edition, 2008, pg 788-789.

9. Itoh, J., Nabeshima, T., & Kameyama, T. (1990). Utility of an elevated plus-maze for the evaluation of memory in mice: effects of nootropics, scopolamine and electroconvulsive shock. Psychopharmacology, 101(1), 27-33.

10. Joel, D. (2006). Current animal models of obsessive compulsive disorder: a critical review. Progress in Neuro-Psychopharmacology and Biological Psychiatry, 30(3), 374-388.

11. Khatri, D. K., & Juvekar, A. R. (2016). Neuroprotective effect of curcumin as evinced by abrogation of rotenone-induced motor deficits, oxidative and mitochondrial dysfunctions in mouse model of Parkinson's disease. Pharmacology Biochemistry and Behavior, 150, 39-47.

12. Lyvia Joao Paulo et al(2005) Behavioural and neurochemical effects on rat of spring after prenatal exposure to alcohol. Neurotoxicology and teratology 27: 585-592.

13. Morris, R. (1984). Developments of a water-maze procedure for studying spatial learning in the rat. Journal of neuroscience methods, 11(1), 47-60.

14. Ohgi, Y., Futamura, T., Kikuchi, T., & Hashimoto, K. (2013). Effects of antidepressants on alternations in serum cytokines and depressive-like behavior in mice after lipopolysaccharide administration. Pharmacology Biochemistry and Behavior, 103(4), 853-859.

15. Porsolt, R. D., Bertin, A., & Jalfre, M. (1977). Behavioral despair in mice: a primary screening test for antidepressants. Archives internationales de pharmacodynamie et de therapie, 229(2), 327-336.

16. Porsolt, R. D., Le Pichon, M., & Jalfre, M. L. (1977). Depression: a new animal model sensitive to antidepressant treatments. Nature, 266(5604), 730.

17. Thiébot, M. H., Martin, P., & Puech, A. J. (1992). Animal behavioural studies in the evaluation of antidepressant drugs. The British Journal of Psychiatry, 160 (Suppl 15), 44-50.

18. S. Pellow, S.E. File, (1985) Validation of open: closed arm entries in an elevated plus-maze as a measure of anxiety in the rat, Journal of neuroscience methods, Volume 14, Issue 3, Pages 149-167.

19. Shoji, H., Hagihara, H., Takao, K., Hattori, S., & Miyakawa, T. (2012). T-maze forced alternation and left-right discrimination tasks for assessing working and reference memory in mice. Journal of visualized experiments: JoVE, (60).

20. Toubas, P. L., Abla, K. A., Cao, W. U., Logan, L. G., & Seale, T. W. (1990). Latency to enter a mirrored chamber: a novel behavioral assay for anxiolytic agents. Pharmacology Biochemistry and Behavior, 35(1), 121-126.

21. Walf, A. A., & Frye, C. A. (2007). The use of the elevated plus maze as an assay of anxiety-related behavior in rodents. Nature protocols, 2(2), 322.

3 EXPERIMENTAL METHODS IN AUTONOMIC PHARMACOLOGY

INTRODUCTION TO AUTONOMIC NERVOUS SYSTEM

The autonomic nervous system (ANS) regulates the body's internal environment. Through regulation of blood pressure, heart rate and strength, respiratory rate and depth, body temperature, and digestive processes, the reflexes of the ANS maintain homeostasis, that is, constant satisfactory conditions for the continuation of vital physiological functions. Although autonomic reflexes have both sensory and motor components, the ANS is technically defined as the motor portion of the reflexes that control and modulate the internal physiological mechanism(s) vital for our continued existence.

The ANS functions largely below the level of consciousness and controls visceral functions. The autonomic nervous system consists of afferent, central and efferent signals. In the case of autonomic afferents, most of the visceral nerves are mixed nerves and are composed of non-myelinated visceral afferent fibers. The cell bodies of these afferent fibers are located in the dorsal root ganglion of spinal nerves and the sensory ganglia (e.g. no dose ganglion of vagus) of cranial nerves. They mediate visceral pain as well as cardiovascular, respiratory and other visceral reflexes. Since, they mediate the cardiovascular reflexes, the ANS could be a potential target in screening of cardiac muscle activities.

In addition, ANS elicits following effects on the target organs

a. Increased heart rate and force of contraction (ionotropic effect) leading to
    1) Increased blood pressure.
    2) Increased stroke volume (more blood is pumped from the heart with each beat).
b. Increased coronary blood flow leading to improved cardiac performance.
c. Increased sweating causing greater cooling of the active body.

d. Dilation of the pupils (mydriasis) presumably to adjust and improve the visibility to adapt to the change in environment.

e. Increased blood flow to the skeletal muscles to enhance effective functioning during duress and/or adverse circumstances.

f. Decreased blood flow to the skin and digestive system to allow shunting in order to increase blood flow to the skeletal muscles.

g. Decreased contractions of the smooth muscles of the urinary bladder and the bowels leading to cessation of urination and defecation. In stressful conditions/ frightening situations (high levels of nor epinephrine released into the hypothalamus and amygdale preventing the central smooth muscle inhibition) leading to urinary incontinence as well as defecation.

As we find the connection of ANS with the cardiac muscles, smooth muscles and skeletal muscles, this system can be used as the potential target in screening pharmacologically active compounds inducing cardiac, smooth or skeletal muscle activities.

Heart is a vital organ and essential to body function. The functioning of the heart depends on various factors like electrolytes and functioning of myocytes.

The myocytes consists of a variety of important membrane systems which generally interact in proximity to produce a series of orchestrated cellular and molecular alterations.

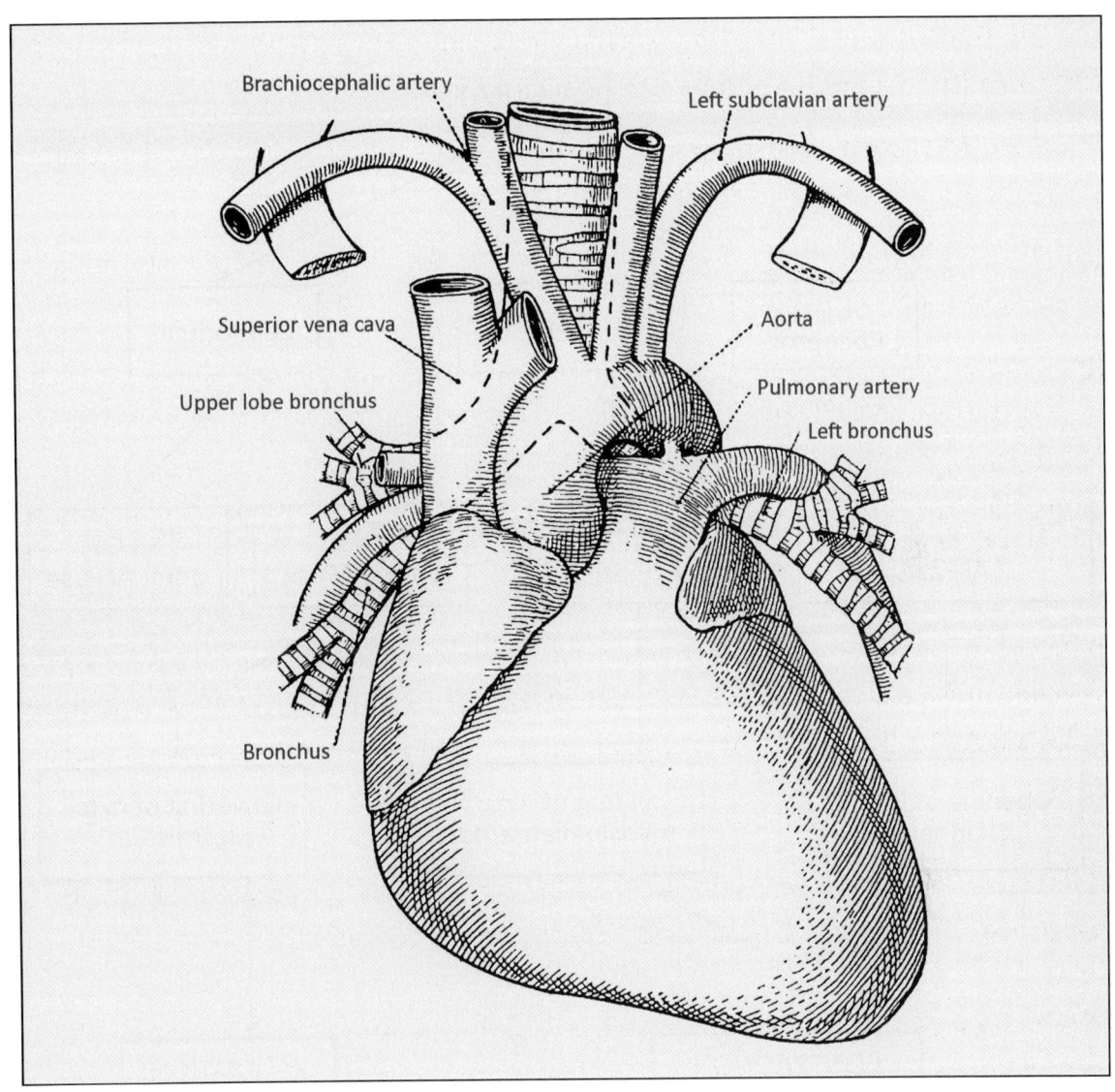

Fig. : Heart

MYOCARDIAL CONTRACTION AND ROLE OF CALCIUM

The importance of Ca^{2+} for the viability of the myocytes has been well recognized for almost a century. Ca^{2+} is important for myocardial metabolism, contractile function, maintaining membrane structure and cellular excitability. This cation in appropriate concentrations is essential for the life of the myocytes. However, in abnormally high or low concentration it is associated with dysfunction and death of myocytes (Dhalla et al., 1981) **(Fig. 3.1 and Fig. 3.2)**.

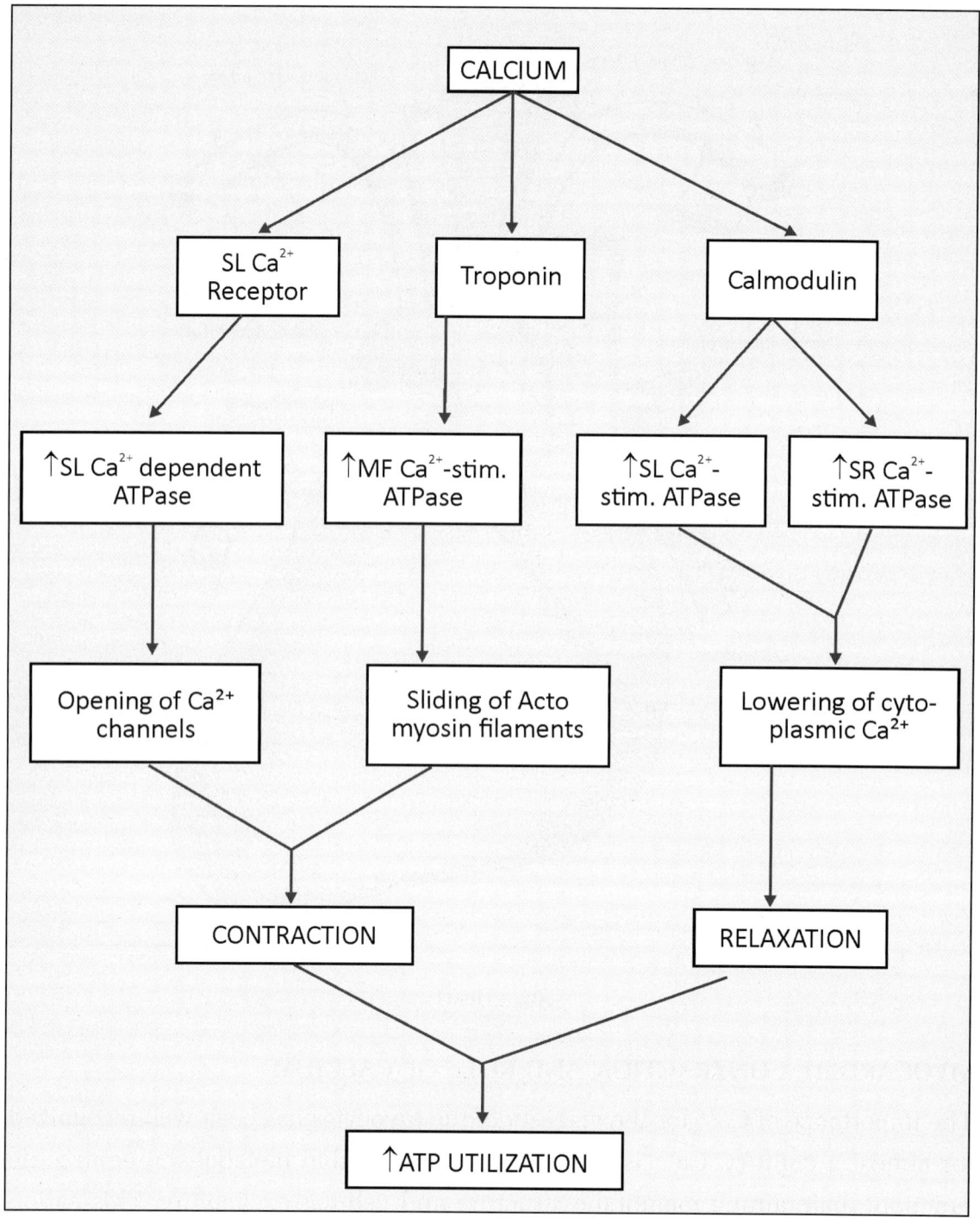

Fig. 3.1: Diagrammatic scheme depicting the interaction of calcium with various receptor proteins activation of various cellular ATPase proteins and the effect on contractile state and energy utilization.

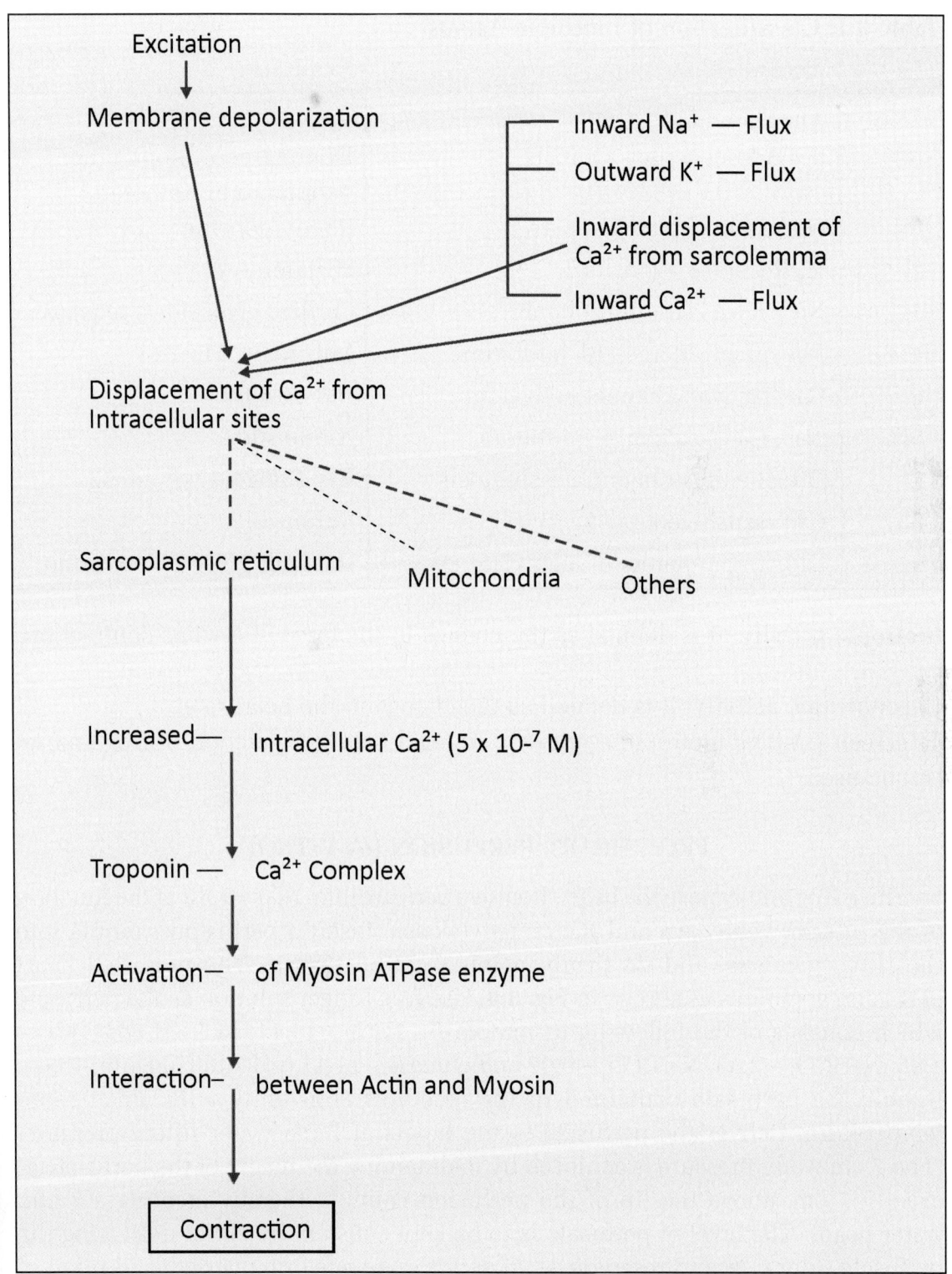

Fig. 3.2: Schematic representation of excitation-contraction coupling in heart muscle

Table 3.1: Classification of Inotropic Agents

Sr. No.	Agents	Examples
1.	The adrenergic agents	
(a)	β_1- Adrenoceptor agonists	Isoproterenol, dopamine, dobutamine, Xamoterol
(b)	α_1-Adrenoceptor agonists	Phenylephrine
2.	H_1-Receptor agonists	Histamine
3.	Na^+, K^+-ATPase Inhibitors	Cardiac glycosides, Quabain
4.	Phosphodiesterase III inhibitors	Milrinone, HL-725
5.	Cardiac Na^+ channel activators	DPI 201-106
6.	Na^+, Ca^{2+} exchange inhibitors	Amiloride
7.	Direct activators of Ca^{2+} channels	Bay K8644, CGP 28392
8.	Ca^{2+} sensitizers	Sulmazole
9.	Direct stimulators of adenylate cyclase	Forskolin, Nor epinephrine

Inotropic activity: It is defined as the change in the force of cardiac contraction.

Chronotropic activity: It is defined as the change in the heart rate.
To screen positive inotropic agents the isolated heart preparation of frog and rat can be used.

FROG HEART PERFUSION (*IN-VITRO*)

Sacrifice frog and expose the heart. Remove pericardium. Make a slit at the junction of the inferior vena cava and the sinus venosus. Insert a perfusion cannula into the sinus venosus, and tie firmly using a cotton thread. The modified heart perfusion apparatus as shown in **Fig. 3.4**. Use frog Ringer solution as the perfusate which consists of the following in mMoles/L. NaCl- 111.11; KCl – 1.88; $CaCl_2$ – 1.08; $NaHCO_3$ – 2.38; NaH_2PO_4 – 0.07 and glucose – 11.11 (pH 7.8)(Guggum, 1953). Bubble the perfusate contained in the reservoir constantly with air at room temperature. Deliver the perfusate to the hearts at 7 cm water filling pressure. (The 7 cm water pressure is achieved by maintaining the height of the perfusate at exactly 7 cm. above the tip of the perfusion cannula thereby creating a 7 cm. water head). The level of perfusate is to be kept constant by either delivering the perfusate from a second reservoir at an appropriate rate or by periodic addition of the Ringer solution to the reservoir.

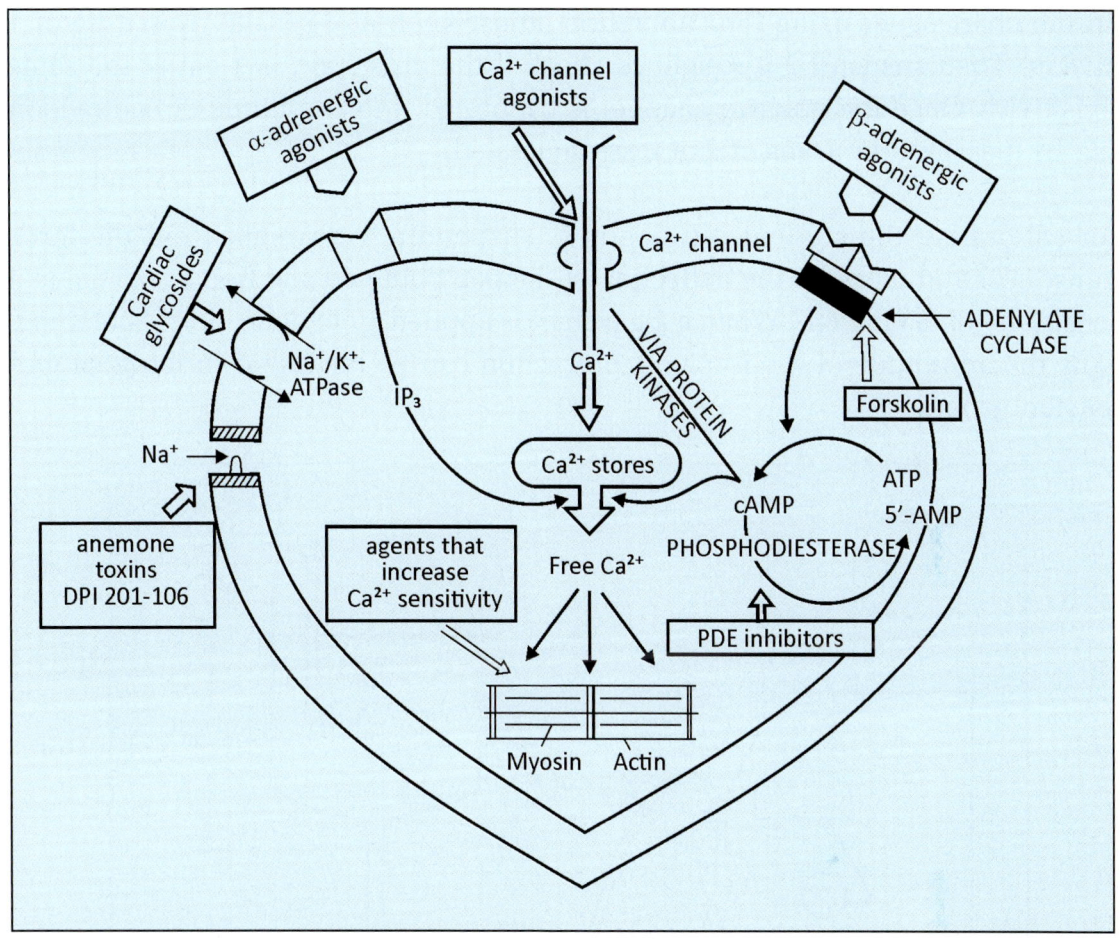

Fig. 3.3: Schematic picture of a myocytes and sites of action of positive inotropic agents.

Monitor the heart rate and the contractile force development by attaching one end of a silk thread to the apex of the heart by means of a palmer clip and the other end of the thread by means to a force displacement transducer after passing it through a pulley. Record the contractile force developed by the heart on a polyrite recorder or student physiograph. At 7 cm water filling pressure and normal Ca^{2+} concentration in the perfusate, the heart develops a contractile force of 1.9 ± 0.5 g. Heart rate varies from one batch of animals to another.

Calibration of the polyrite and the student physiograph

Connect the force displacement transducer to the polyrite channel to be calibrated and expose to a 1 g weight and adjust the corresponding pen deflection to 0.5 cm on the chart paper using the calibration adjust knob at a sensitivity setting of 1 mv/cm. Then suspend 2 g weight to check if the deflection is 1 cm at the same sensitivity. Once the polyrite channel is calibrated, the amplitude of contraction can be measured in terms of g of force generated.

For calibrating the student physiograph, suspend a 1 g weight from the force transducer and measure the deflection of the pen obtained and find as 0.5 cm at a sensitivity of 0.5 mv/cm. When a 2 g weight is applied 1 cm deflection is obtained. Now the amplitude of the force of contraction can be measured in terms of g of tension generated.

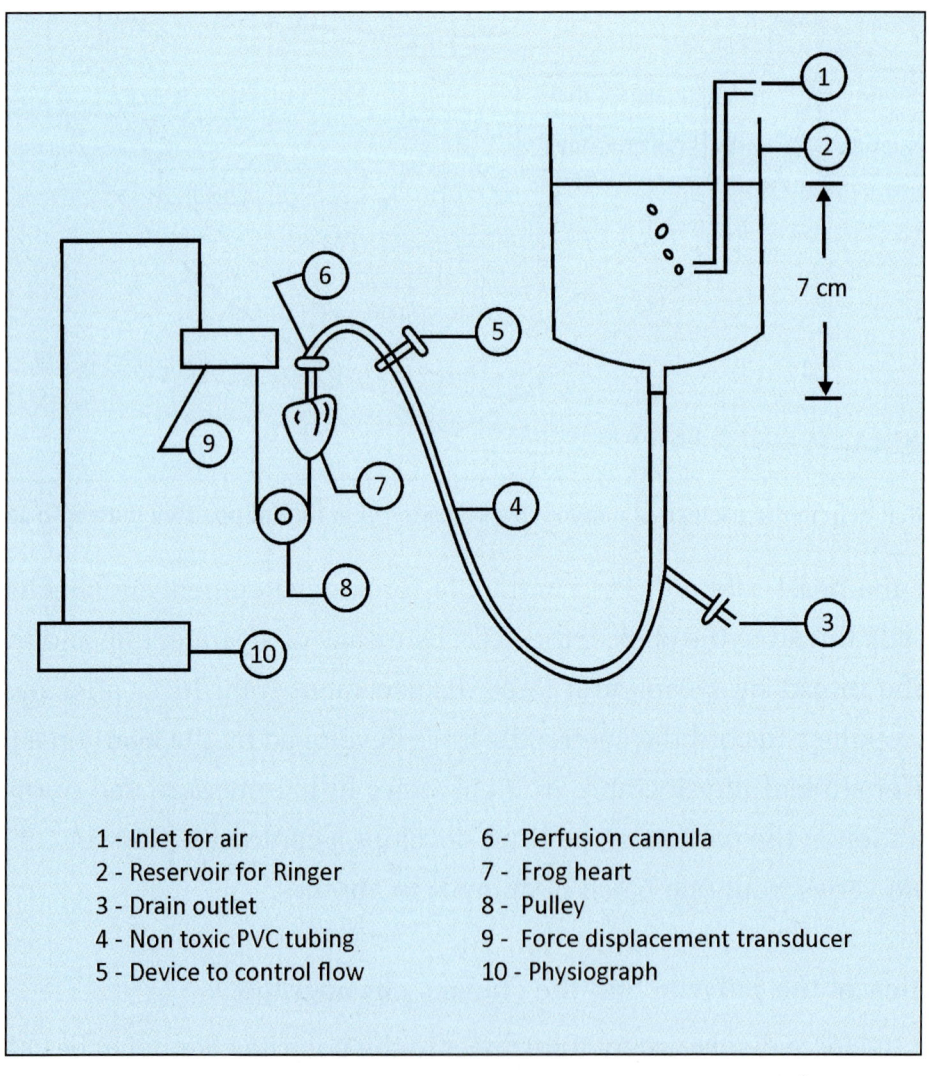

7 cm

1 - Inlet for air
2 - Reservoir for Ringer
3 - Drain outlet
4 - Non toxic PVC tubing
5 - Device to control flow

6 - Perfusion cannula
7 - Frog heart
8 - Pulley
9 - Force displacement transducer
10 - Physiograph

Fig. 3.4: Set up for isolated frog heart.

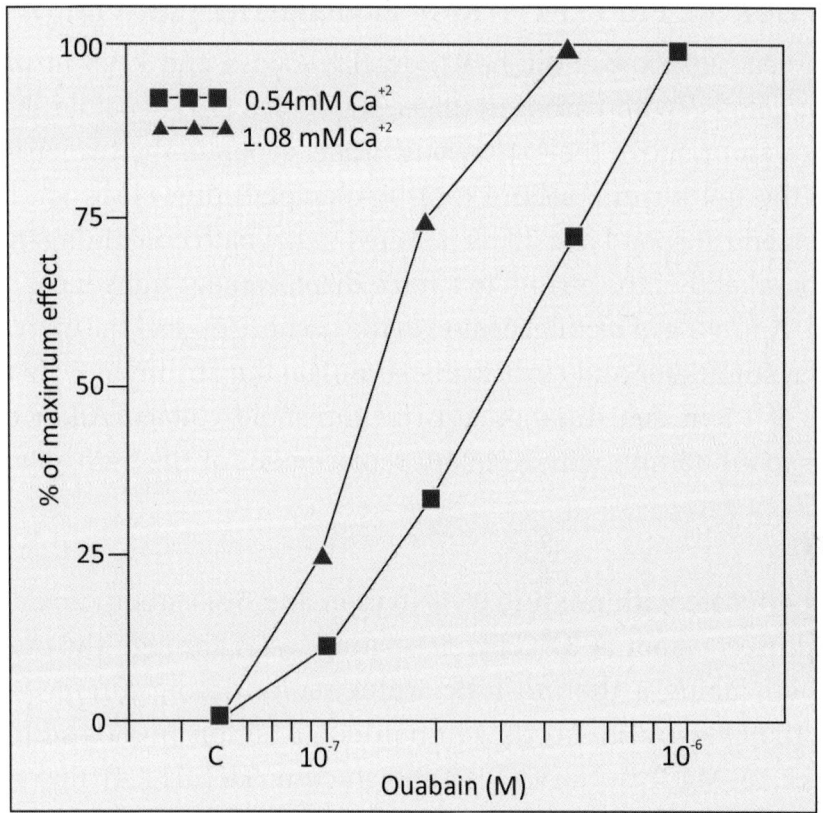

Fig. 3.5: Effect of Ouabain on frog heart at different calcium levels.

Effect of ouabain on isolated frog heart at different
Ca^{2+} concentrations

The 'X' axis represents the molar concentration of
ouabain.

Y-axis represents the percent of maximum effect.

Each point represents the mean of six determinations.
Vertical bars represent standard error of the mean.

Fig. 3.6: Effect of Ouabain on isolated frog heart at different Ca^{2+} concentrations.

GUINEA PIG LEFT ATRIAL PREPARATION (*IN-VITRO*)

Sacrifice guinea pig. Expose the heart, quickly excise and keep in physiological salt solution aerated with carbogen (95% CO_2 + 5% O_2). Separate the atria from the ventricles and remove the extraneous tissue, separate the two atria from each other. Take the left atrium, secure to a bipolar platinum electrode through the apical margin and suspend in a 20 ml jacketed organ bath containing the perfusate. Attach the basal end of the atrium to a force displacement transducer by means of a silk thread. Apply 1 g of resting tension to the tissue. Connect the bipolar platinum electrode to a stimulator and electrically stimulate the atrium to 1 Hz with square wave pulses of 1.5 m. sec. duration at twice threshold voltage. Allow the tissue to stabilize for about 30 min with frequent replacement of the perfusate.

The perfusate

Bubble the perfusate with mixture 95% oxygen and 5% carbon dioxide; maintain the temperature constant at 37°C by circulating water through the outer jacket of the organ bath using a thermostatic water recirculating pump. Under these conditions, the Chenoweth-koelle solution composition (mMoles/L): NaCl: 135, KCl:5, $CaCl_2$:2.18, $MgCl_2$:2, $NaHCO_3$:19 and glucose: 9.9 (pH 7.4). Record Left atrial contractions on a student physiograph and express the tension developed in g. The left atria develop a mean force of about 0.5 ± 0.03g (Chenoweth-Koelle, 1946).

Administration of drugs

Drugs are administered as bolus injections or by adding to the perfusate or by continuous infusion. When drugs are administered by adding to the perfusion medium the dose response curves are performed in a cumulative fashion, each time taking into consideration the amount of drug already present in the perfusate. Force measurements are made after peak responses are developed. In most cases, it is either 5 or 10 min after addition of the drug. Only in case of some specific drugs it is 15-20 min after the addition of the drug. Bolus injections are made at a fixed point on the tubing above the perfusion cannula and the volume of bolus injections are kept constant at 1.0 ml throughout the study. Continuous infusion of the drug is achieved using a continuous slow injector pump. Drugs are infused at a rate of 1 ml/min throughout the study. During infusion the drug solution is introduced at a fixed point above the heart to maintain the constant filling pressure.

MEASUREMENT OF INOTROPIC EFFECT IN GUINEA PIG LEFT ATRIA (*IN-VITRO*)

Experiments are performed on the guinea pigs of either sex having body weight in the range of 300 to 400 g. Guinea pigs are sacrificed. The left atria is rapidly isolated from the heart of animal and placed in 20 ml organ bath containing Chenoweth-Koelle solution (Composition mentioned in the previous experiment). A resting tension of 1 g is applied to tissue. The atrium is electrically stimulated to 1 Hz with square wave pulses of 1.5 m/sec duration at twice threshold voltage by bipolar platinum electrode connected to a stimulator. Left atrial contractions are recorded on a student's physiograph through force displacement transducer and the tension developed is expressed in g. In the guinea pig left atrial experiements drug is administered via perfusate. Contractions of the atria are recorded after the peak response is developed.

STATISTICAL ANALYSIS

All the experiments are repeated six times and the values expressed as mean ± sem. Statistical evaluation are performed by using the student's 't' test for paired values. A 'P' value $P < 0.05$ was considered significant.

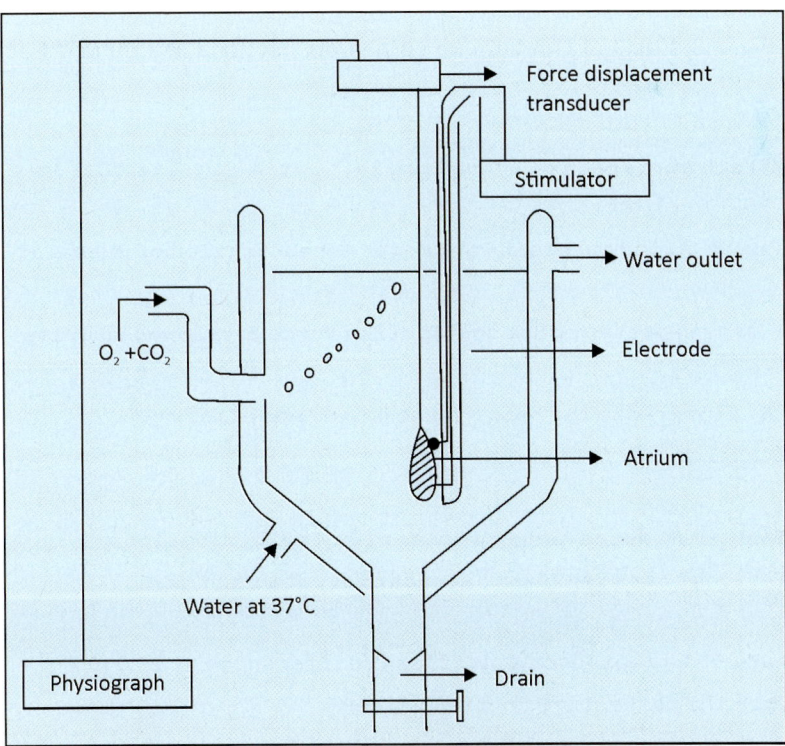

Fig. 3.7: Set-up for isolated guinea-pig left atrium.

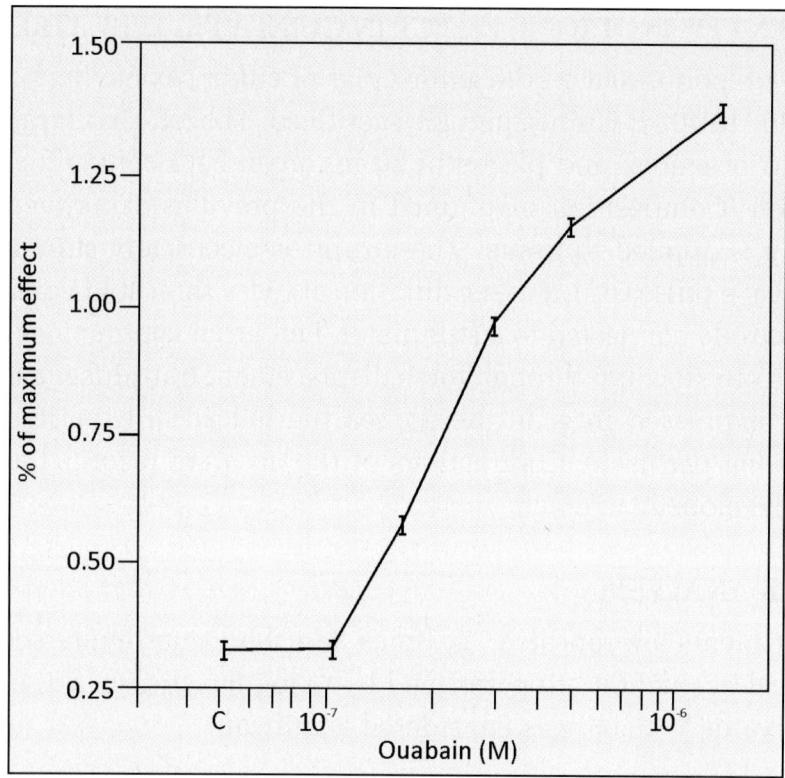

Fig. 3.8: Effect of Ouabain on guinea pig left atria at 1.09 mM Ca^{2+}

Effect of ouabain on guinea pig left atria at 1.09 mM Ca^{2+} level.

The 'X' axis represents the molar concentration of ouabain.

Y-axis represents the contractile force developed in grams.

'C' represents the basal force developed prior to ouabain administration.

Each point represents the mean of six determinations.
Vertical bars represent standard error of the mean.

Asterisks represent significant differences at $P < 0.05$ from the respective control values.

Fig. 3.9: Effect of Ouabain on guinea pig left atria at 1.09 mM Ca^{2+} level.

WORKING HEART APPARATUS (LANGENDORFF HEART PREPARATION)

The working heart apparatus used in this study is a modified version of neely's Original working heart apparatus (Neely et al. 1967) as described by Vadlamudi et. al. (1982).

The working heart apparatus as shown in **Fig. 3.10**, consists of a jacketed primary and a jacketed filling reservoir. The primary reservoir is connected through a 3-way stop cock to a 15 gauge steel aortic cannula. The primary reservoir that is connected to the aortic cannula is situated 45 cms above the aortic cannula. The other end of the 3-way stop cock is connected to a filling reservoir. The filling reservoir is connected to a 16 gauge stell perfusion cannula and the reservoir is fixed such that it can be moved up and down in steps to provide various filling pressures. Perfusate level in the jacketed reservoir is maintained at a constant level. The aortic cannula is connected to a external peripheral resistance by means of another 3-way stopcock. The external peripheral resistance consists of polyethylene (PE) 160 tubing with a 1 ml air cushion. The perfusate is maintained at 37°C by means of a constant – temperature water recirculating pump (Siskin-Julabo, Model V12B). The perfusate in the reservoir is also constantly aerated with a mixture of 95% oxygen and 5% carbon dioxide. The perfusate used is the one described previously by Chenoweth and Koelle (1946). This Chenoweth-Koelle solution contained the following in millimolar quantities: NaCl, 120; KCl, 5.6; $CaCl_2$, 2.18; $MgCl_2$, 2.1; $NaHCO_3$, 19; glucose, 9.9 and EDTA, 0.03. When aerated with 95% O_2 – 5% CO_2 mixture at 37°C, the pH of the solution is maintained at 7.4.

SCHEMATIC REPRESENTATION OF WORKING HEART APPARATUS (LANGENDORFF HEART PREPARATION)

The set up consists of a jacketed primary reservoir (1) and a jacketed filling reservoir (2). The primary reservoir is connected through a three way stop-cock (7) to a 15 gauge steel aortic cannula (3) or to a filling reservoir. The filling reservoir is connected to a 16 gauge steel left atrial cannula (4). The primary reservoir that is connected to the aortic cannula is situated 45 cm above the cannula. The filling reservoir can be moved up or down in steps to provide various filing pressures between 5-22.5 cm of H_2O. The aortic cannula is connected to an external peripheral resistance of 75 cm polyethylene tubing (5) and a 1 ml syringe (6). The perfusate in the reservoir is constantly aerated through the oxygenator and is maintained at 37°C by means of a constant temperature water recicrculating pump.

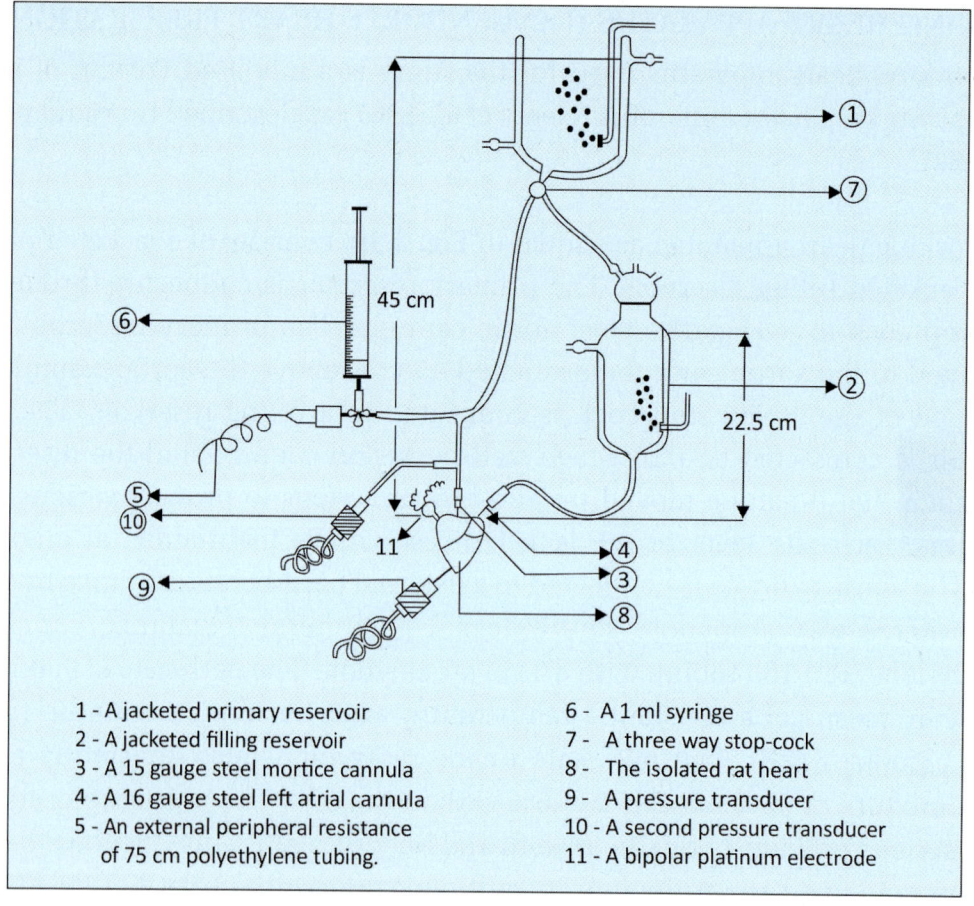

1 - A jacketed primary reservoir
2 - A jacketed filling reservoir
3 - A 15 gauge steel mortice cannula
4 - A 16 gauge steel left atrial cannula
5 - An external peripheral resistance
    of 75 cm polyethylene tubing.

6 - A 1 ml syringe
7 - A three way stop-cock
8 - The isolated rat heart
9 - A pressure transducer
10 - A second pressure transducer
11 - A bipolar platinum electrode

Fig. 3.10: Schematic representation of working heart apparatus (Neely et al., 1967).

The isolated rat heart (8) is attached to the aortic cannula through the aorta and perfused initially in the retrograde manner at 45 cm water filing pressure. The left ventricular chamber is connected to a pressure transducer. The left atrium is cannulated with the atrial cannula and the perfusion is switched to the working mode. In the working heart mode, perfusate from filling reservoir entered the left ventricular chamber, pumped out through the aorta into the peripheral resistance. The second pressure transducer (10) was used to record the intra-aortic pressure. The heart is paced, by placing a bipolar platinum electrode (11) on the left atrium at 300 beats/minute. The volume of the perfusate coming out against the peripheral resistance is measured and is considered to be the aortic output **(Fig. 3.10)**.

HEART PERFUSION AND DETERMINATION OF THE CARDIAC FUNCTION

Once the apparatus is made ready for regular experimentation, the animals are sacrificed. The hearts are quickly removed and are placed in Chenoweth-koelle buffer maintained at 37°C. All the extraneous tissue are freed, and after locating the aortic stump the hearts are attached to the 15 gauge aortic cannula through the aortic stump and the perfusion is started in the retrograde fashion. The hearts are allowed to get perfused for some time. The remnants of the pulmonary vein are located and a 16 gauge left atrial filling cannula is inserted into the left atrium through the pulmonary vein and tied. The retrograde perfusion is stopped and working heart mode is initiated to estimate the cardiac workload. A polythene tube (PE 90) of length 3 cm is inserted through apex of the heart in to the left ventricle and the other end of the PE tubing is attached to a pressure transducer to measure the left ventricular pressure development (LVPD). In the working mode the perfusate from left atrium enters the left ventricle and then it is pumped out into the aortic stump. To the aortic stump which now leads to an external peripheral resistance, a second pressure transducer is attached through a side arm to measure the intra-aortic pressure. Aortic and LVPD are recorded on a Medicare polyrite/ student physiograph.

The hearts are electrically stimulated by placing a bipolar electrode on the left atrium. The hearts are stimulated at 300 beats/min. with pulses of 5 msec. duration and twice threshold voltage from a stimulator.

The hearts are allowed to stabilize at 15 cm H_2O filling pressure for 15 min. The LVPD value at 15 cm atrial filling pressure (AFP) was around 160 mm Hg.

The cardiac function obtained is expressed as LVPD, rate of rise of pressure +dP/dt (contraction), and rate of decline of pressure –dP/dt, (relaxation).

dP/dt is calculated manually by drawing a tangent line to the pressure trace at the point of maximum slope. The slope of this line is normally calculated by constructing a right angle triangle by dropping a vertical and drawing a horizontal back to the tangent line. However, as the recording system used is curvilinear, this method is modified slightly. It is assumed that the maximum positive slope of the pressure curve occurred at approximately 25 mm Hg and the negative slope at 75 mm Hg. At these deflections the recording pen is about 6° and 2° respectively from the horizontal. Therefore to correct this, the constructed right angled triangles are also titled at 6° or 2° as shown in **Fig. 3.11**.

Determination of positive and negative dP/dt from left ventricular pressure trace

Tangent lines (2 and 3) are drawn to the left ventricular pressure trace (1) at the points of maximum slope, which are approximately at 25 mm Hg for the pressure curve. Slopes of these tangents are calculated by constructing right angled triangles by dropping verticals (4 and 5) and drawing horizontals back to tangents lines. Since the recording pen is about 6° at 25 mm Hg and 2° at 75 mm Hg from the horizontal, the right angled triangles A and b are titled by 6° and 2° respectively. The slope is calculated from the formula:

$$\text{Slope of the hypotenuse} = \frac{\text{Opposite side}}{\text{Adjacent side}} \quad \text{or} \quad \frac{\text{Vertical}}{\text{Horizontal}}$$

Vertical can be converted to pressure (mm Hg) from chart Calibration and horizontal to time (sec) from chart speed.

$$\text{Then slope} = \frac{\text{mm Hg}}{\text{sec}}$$

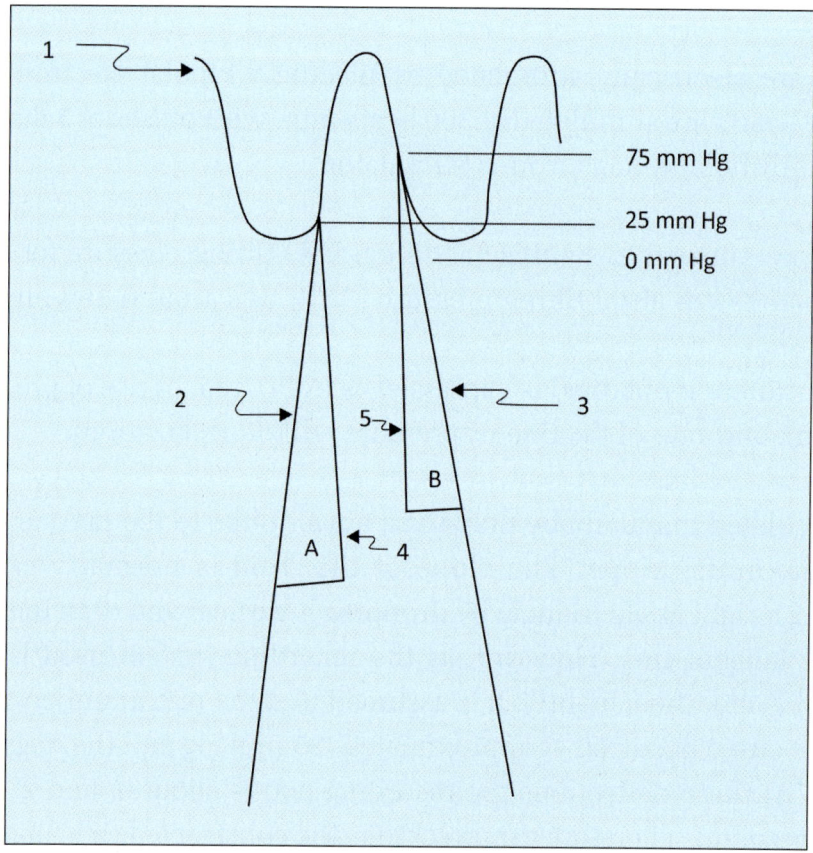

Fig. 3.11: The right angled triangle.

Effect of 70 cm water column as afterload.

Left ventricular pressure development at various left atrial filling pressures in isolated perfused working hearts from control rats.

All the values are expressed as the mean ± S.E.M. Numbers in parentheses are the number of animals used. LVDP or left ventricular developed pressure is expressed as mm Hg on the Y-axis. Left atrial filling pressure is expressed as cm H_2O on the X-axis.

Fig. 3.12: Effect of 70 cm water column as afterload.

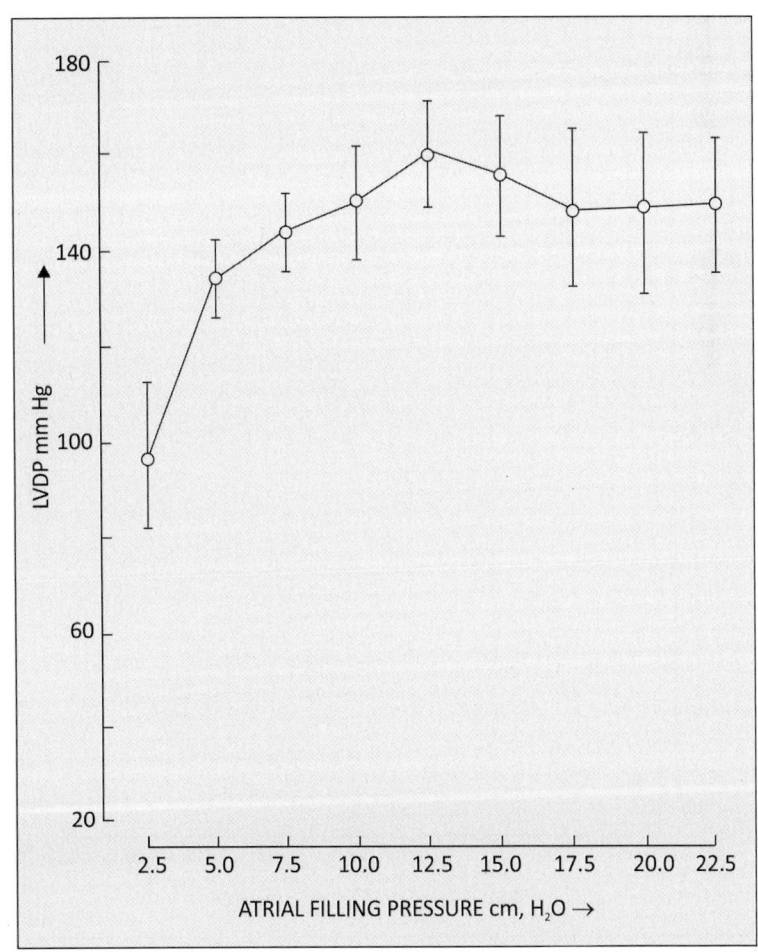

Fig. 3.13: LVDP Vs Atrial filling pressure.

Effect of 55 cm PE tubing as afterload.

Left ventricular pressure development at various left atrial filling pressures in isolated perfused working hearts from control rats.

All the values are expressed as the mean $\pm$ S.E.M. Numbers in parentheses are the number of animals used. LVDP or left ventricular developed pressure is expressed as mm Hg on the Y-axis. Left atrial filling pressure is expressed as cm H_2O on the X-axis.

Fig. 3.14: Effect of 55 cm PE tubing as afterload.

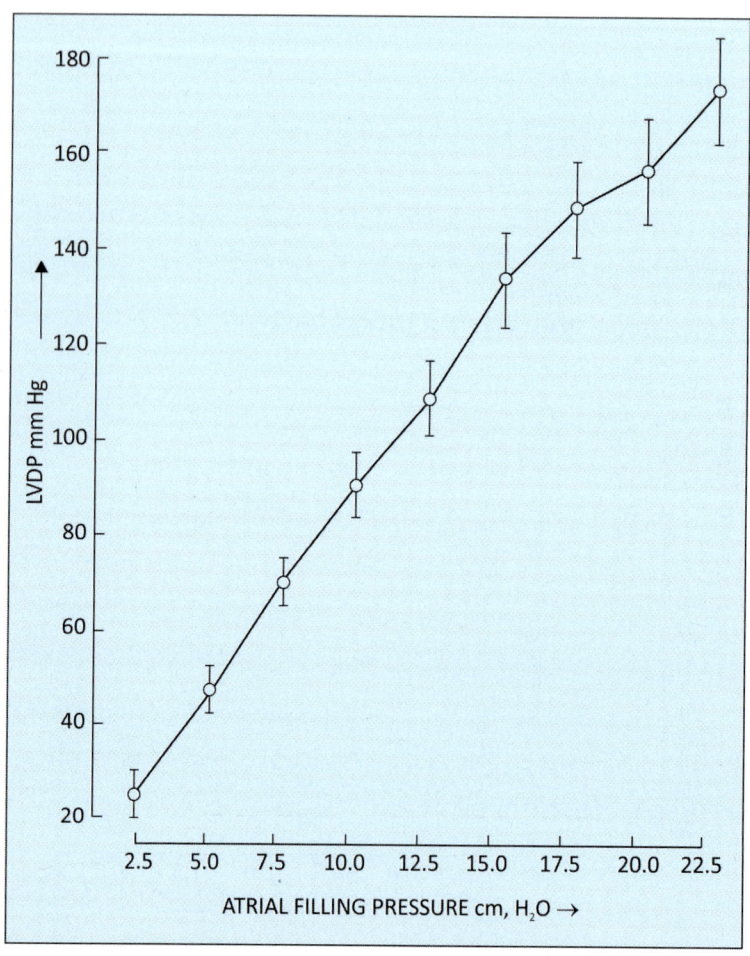

Fig. 3.15: LVPD v/s Atrial filling pressure.

ISOLATED MUSCLE

Introduction

Isolated muscle preparations have been very convenient and valuable pharmacological tool, for evaluating drug receptor interactions and recording activity of tissues as against various concentrations of drugs, acting at specific receptors present on them. Isolated muscle experiments come with the advantage of simplicity, versatility and reproducibility. We can obtain large number of preparations from single animal and comparatively small amount of drug is needed as against intact animal. Moreover in isolated muscle experiments, the physiological factors like absorption, distribution, metabolism, excretion of drugs, and nerve reflexes do not interfere with the response of test drugs.

Benefits of testing drug effect on isolated muscle

Isolated muscle offers advantage over *in-vivo* testing to assessing the direct effect of drug and avoid variables that may happens during intact animal experiments. Isolated muscle also enables an improved analysis of a dose–response relationship, without the adverse side effects which may be seen during *in-vivo* work. During such *in-vitro* studies, a target muscle(s) is isolated, usually from an experimental animal mostly rodent/amphibian, and placed in an organ bath which is perfused with suitable physiological salt solution such as Tyrode or Krebs-Henseleit or Ringer solution (high in glucose and contains other essential salts to mimic blood plasma) and aerated.

The primary advantage of isolated tissue experimental technique is that the tissue is living and functions as a whole tissue, with a physiological outcome (contraction or relaxation) that is relevant to the body. It involves events such as drug-receptor interaction, signal transduction, second messenger generation, change in smooth muscle excitability, and change in tissue function. While other techniques allow study of each of these events (e.g. radioligand binding for drug-receptor affinity, measurement of second messengers), the isolated tissue bath technique allows for integration of all these steps in a single response.

Table 3.2: Summary of major receptors expressed on various tissues, their agonists and antagonists

Smooth Muscles				
Tissue	**Physiological Solution**	**Receptors present**	**Drug**	
			Agonists	**Antagonists**
Guinea pig ileum	Tyrode	Histaminergic	Histamine	Mepyramine Cimetidine
		Cholinergic	Acetylcholine	Atropine Pirenzepine
		Serotonergic	5-HT	Ketanserine
Guinea Pig Tracheal Chain	Krebs	Adrenergic Histaminergic	Adrenaline, Histamine	Phentolamine Mepyramine
Rat colon	Tyrode	Adrenergic	Adrenaline Noradrenaline	Phentolamine Phentolamine
Rat fundus	Krebs	Serotonergic Cholinergic	5-HT Acetylcholine	Ketanserine Atropine Pirenzepine
		Histaminergic	Histamine	Mepyramine
Rat uterus	De Jalon	Oxytocic Serotonergic Adrenergic	Oxytocin 5-HT Adrenaline	Atosiban Ketanserine Phentolamine
Rat anococcygeus	Krebs	Muscarinic α-adrenergic Serotonergic	Acetylcholine Noradrenaline 5-HT	Atropine Phentolamine Ketanserine
Rat ascending colon	Tyrode	Adrenergic Muscarinic	Noradrenaline Acetylcholine	Phentolamine Atropine Pirenzepine
		Serotonergic	5-HT	Ketanserine
Rat descending colon	Tyrode	Muscarinic	Acetylcholine	Atropine
Skeletal Muscles				
Tissue	**Physiological Solution**	**Receptors present**	**Drug**	
			Agonists	**Antagonists**
Frog rectus abdominis	Frog Ringer	Nicotinic	Acetylcholine	d-tubocurarine Succinylcholine
Leech dorsal muscle	Frog-ringer or Locke's solution	Nicotinic	Acetylcholine	d-tubocurarine Succinylcholine

GUINEA PIG ILEUM

Guinea Pig ileum is most sensitive to histamine and also responds to other spasmogens like Acetylcholine, Serotonin, Bradykinin and Angiotensin (Ghosh, 2015). It has the spontaneous activity and specificity is improved by using atropine (for histamine assay) or mepyramine (for acetylcholine) in tyrode.

Protocol for separation of tissue and sample handling

For isolation of ileum healthy guinea pig (200-400 g) is sacrificed following ethical norms and the animal is exsanguinated. The abdomen is cut opened by giving midline incision and the caecum is identified. Caecum is lifted upward in order to identify ileocaecal junction. The portion of ileum remaining after leaving 10 cm from the ileocaecal junction is taken. This is because the initial portion near ileocaecal junction contain excitatory α-adrenoceptors (Munro, 1953). The isolated ileum is cleaned by allowing slow flow of Tyrode solution into lumen.

Guinea pig ileum preparation

Mesentery are carefully removed and the tissue is cleaned of fats. The lumen is thoroughly cleaned by passing PSS slowly through it multiple times with the help of pipette. Care should be taken not to allow excessive stretching of the tissue while cleaning. Nearly 1.5-2 cm long piece of tissue is the transferred to Petri dish containing freshly prepared Tyrode solution. Diagonally opposite ends of the tissue are tied to two separate threads by passing fine sewing needle through the gut and ensuring the lumen remains open. One thread is tied to the lower end of aeration tube and transferred carefully into the organ tube containing physiological salt solution. The upper end of the tissue preparation is tied to the frontal writing lever which is balanced and adjusted for optimum magnification. A load (working load) of 1-1.5 g is attached to the writing arm of the lever at equidistance from fulcrum **(Fig. 3.17)**. Contact time of 30-60 seconds is maintained for recording tissue response.

Therapeutic relevance

The preparation is most commonly used for performing bioassay of histamine, acetylcholine, serotonin and their respective antagonists.

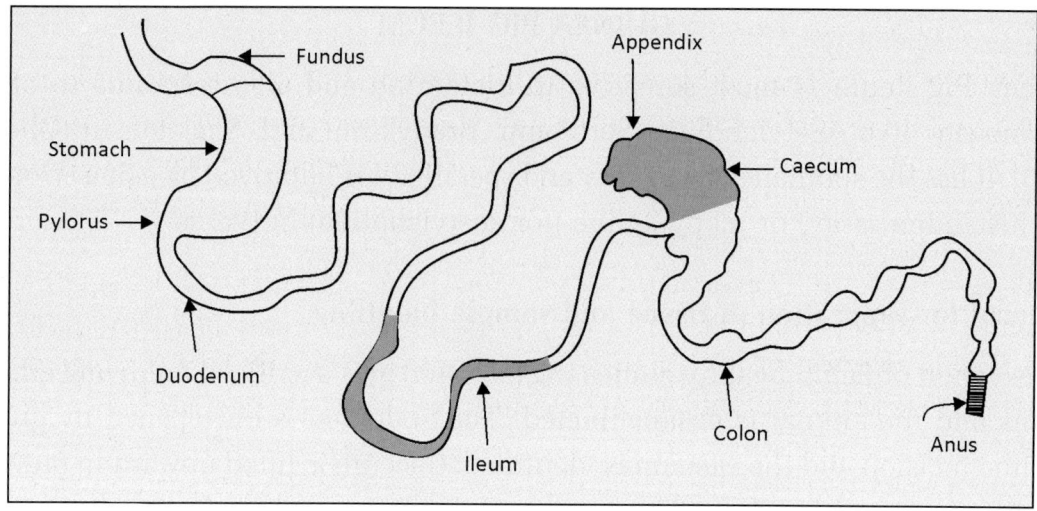

Fig. 3.16: Schematic of gastrointestinal tract.

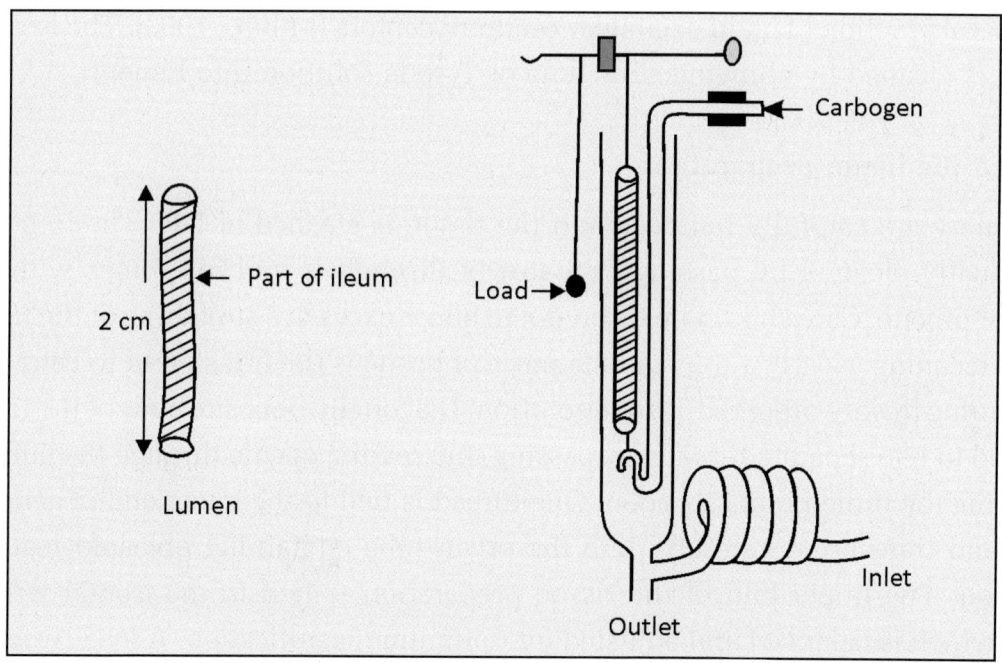

Fig. 3.17: Mounting of guinea pig ileum.

GUINEA PIG TRACHEAL CHAIN

Protocol for separation of tissue and sample handling

Adult Guinea-pig weighing 300-600 g is sacrificed following all ethical norms. The tracheal tube from the cervical portion, approximately 2 cm inferior to the larynx is removed and immediately placed in cool Krebs solution.

Guinea pig tracheal chain preparations

Isolated trachea is cleaned by removing the surrounding connective tissues until a glistering white cartilaginous surface is observed. The tissue also includes a strip of smooth muscle on the posterior side. The trachea is opened by cutting the cartilaginous part vertically in the midline. Subsequently, it is also cut into transverse strips each of which contains a central segment of smooth muscle with cartilage at the ends. Tracheal strips are joined end to end and a tracheal chain is prepared. Tracheal chain is then mounted in a student organ bath, and perfused with Kreb's solution at 37°C and solution aerated (bubbling with oxygen). For recording responses, isotonic frontal writing lever precisely balanced for a tension of 0.5 g, and tracheal chain is allowed to relax for 60-90 minutes. Tissue responses to drug are recorded by maintaining contact period of 90-120 sec and recovery period of 20 minutes. (Castillo, 1948).

Therapeutic relevance

It is employed for studying effects of bronchodilators like adrenaline, isopranaline. These drugs inhibit the contractions induced by histamine.

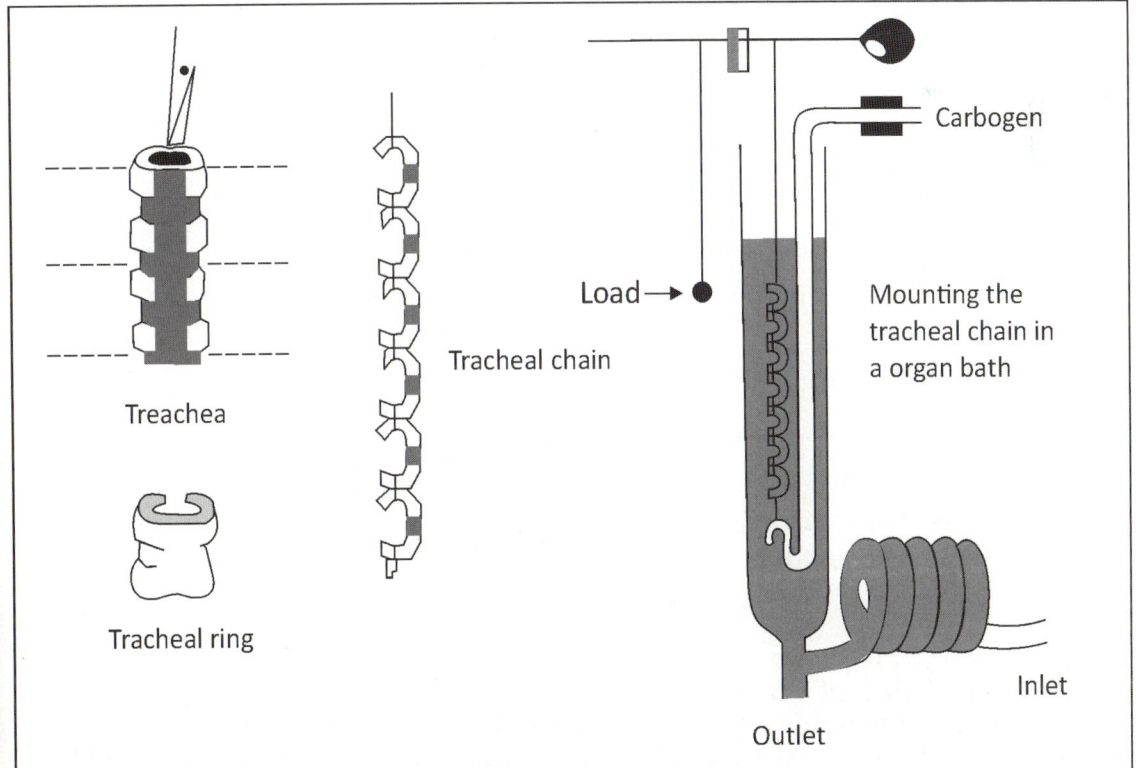

Fig. 3.18: Preparation and mounting of guinea pig tracheal chain

Anatomy of Rat gastrointestinal tract

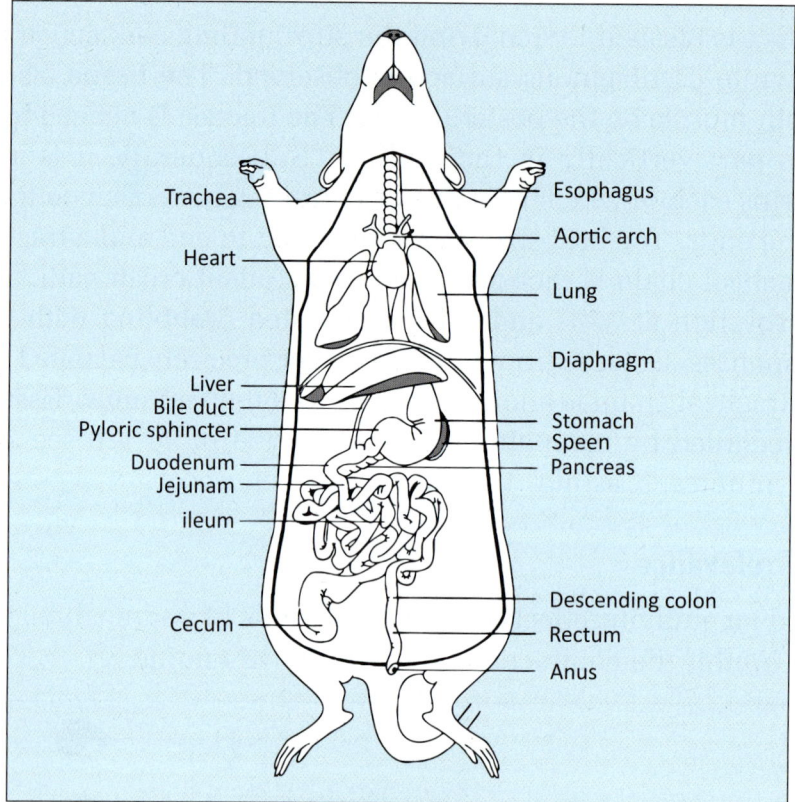

Fig. 3.19: Anatomy of rat.

RAT COLON

The rat colon can be divided into 3 regions (proximal, distal, and cecum) both morphologically and functionally (Ferre and Ruckebusch, 1985).

Protocol for separation of tissue

Overnight fasted male or female rat is sacrificed following all ethical norms. Abdomen is cut opened and colon which is immediately attached to the caecum is located. The colon is rapidly removed and placed in a petri-dish containing Tyrode solution. For studies using rat colon normally proximal 4 cm portion is used.

Sample preparation of rat colon

About 4 cm long segment of colon is taken and cut into longitudinal strips (20 mm × 4 mm). The strip is then suspended in organ bath containing Tyrode solution at 31°C. This solution is aerated with carbogen (5% CO_2: 95% O_2) to maintain the pH of the solution between 7.3 and 7.4. The preparations is allowed to equilibrate in the Tyrode solution for at least 30 min prior to experiment.

For achieving enhanced sensitivity to noradrenaline and to reduce spontaneous activity, the tissue can be stored at 4°C for 24 hours.

Therapeutic relevance

Rat colon serves as a valuable tissue preparation for studying effect of Noradrenaline, substance P and adrenaline. Other drugs to which rat colon is sensitive to some extent include angiotensin and $PGF_{2\alpha}$.

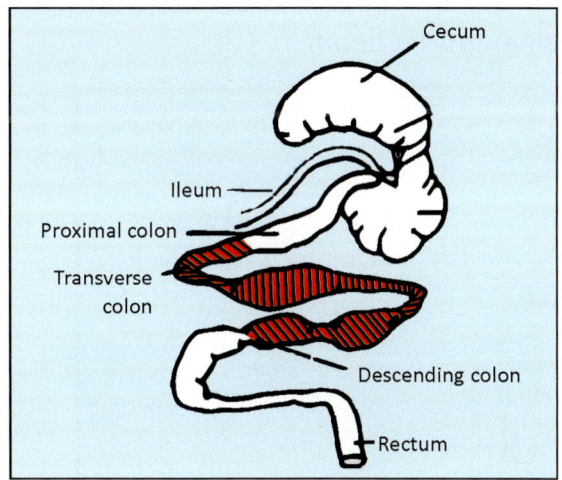 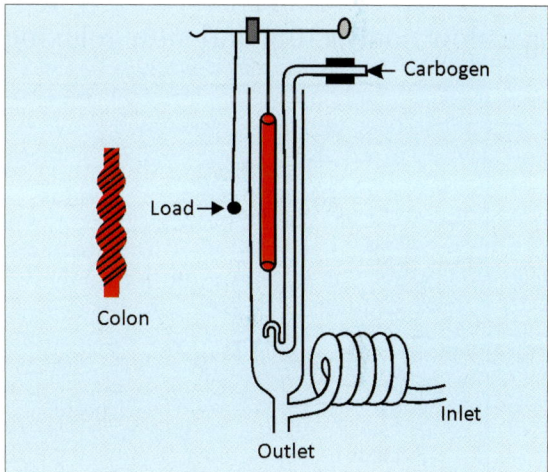

Fig. 3.20: Rat colon and mounting of rat colon strip.

RAT FUNDUS

Protocol for separation of tissue

A healthy male or female rat weighing 200-300 g is killed by following all ethical norms. The abdomen is cut open immediately and stomach is located. The whole stomach is rapidly dissected out and kept in Kreb's solution.

Sample preparations of rat fundus

The stomach contents are washed off and stomach is opened along lesser curvature. Stomach is then placed on a cork mat soaked in salt solution. The upper portion of stomach which appears gray in color is called fundus. Fundus part is isolated from body of the stomach. The preparation is then placed in a petri dish containing Kreb's solution.

A strip is isolated and alternate transverse cuts are made in order to preserve the longitudinal muscles. A cotton thread is tied on both ends of the strip and the preparation is mounted in organ bath containing Kreb's solution at 37°C. The tissue is equilibrated for 90 minutes and responses are recorded keeping the contact time 90 seconds.

Therapeutic relevance

Rat fundus is a sensitive tissue for studying the agonistic action of acetylcholine (ACh), 5-hydroxy-tryptamine (5-HT), histamine and bradykinin. This preparation is a slow contracting and slow relaxing tissue unlike ileum.

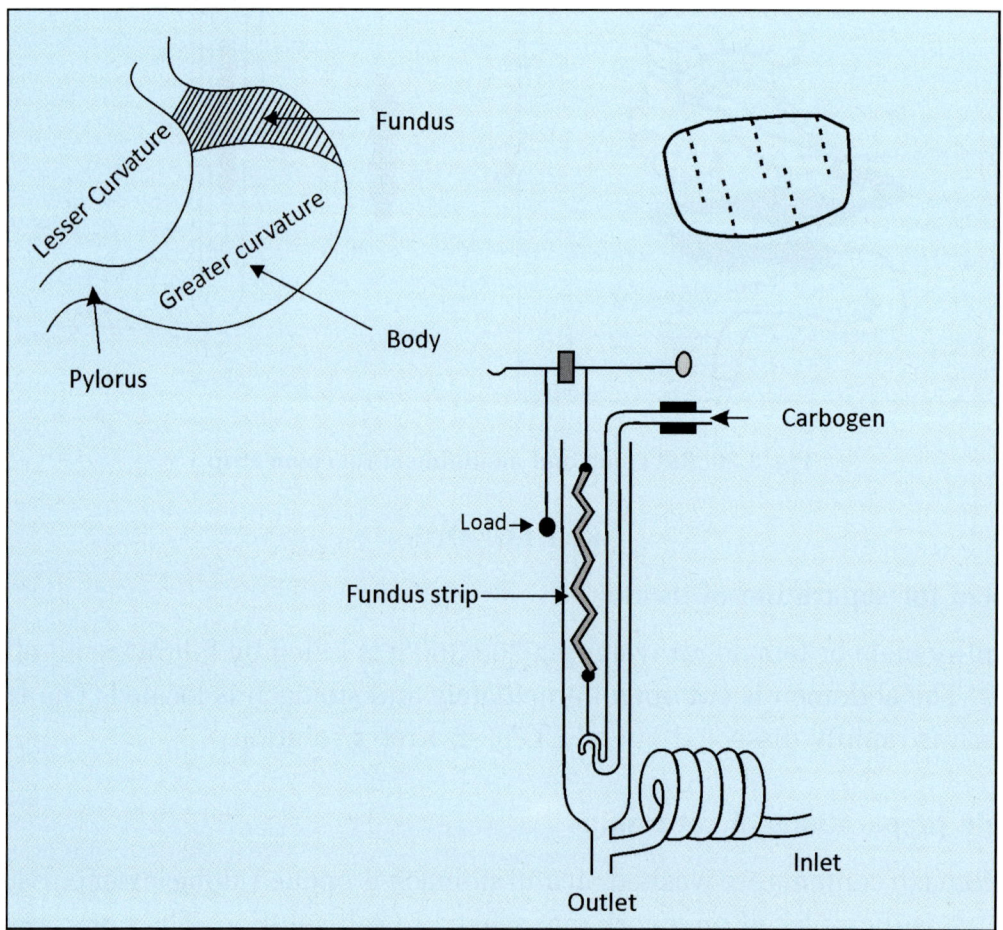

Fig. 3.21: Preparation and mounting of rat fundus strip.

RAT UTERUS

Protocol for separation of tissue

A virgin female rat weighing 150-200 g is injected with diethylstilbestrol at a dose 0.1 mg/100 g body weight for increasing sensitivity and obtaining a relatively stable tissue preparation. After 24 hours of stilbesterol injection rat is sacrificed following all ethical norms. The abdomen is cut opened and uterus is located.

For performing serotonin assay diethylstilbestrol is given at a higher dose of 0.25 mg/100g for three days before sacrificing the animal (Ghosh, 2015).

Sample preparation of rat uterus

The uterus is located and uterine horns are quickly dissected out. Both uterine horns are transferred to a petri-dish containing De-Jalon's solution. The uterine horns are cleaned of attached adipose tissue and one of them is taken for mounting

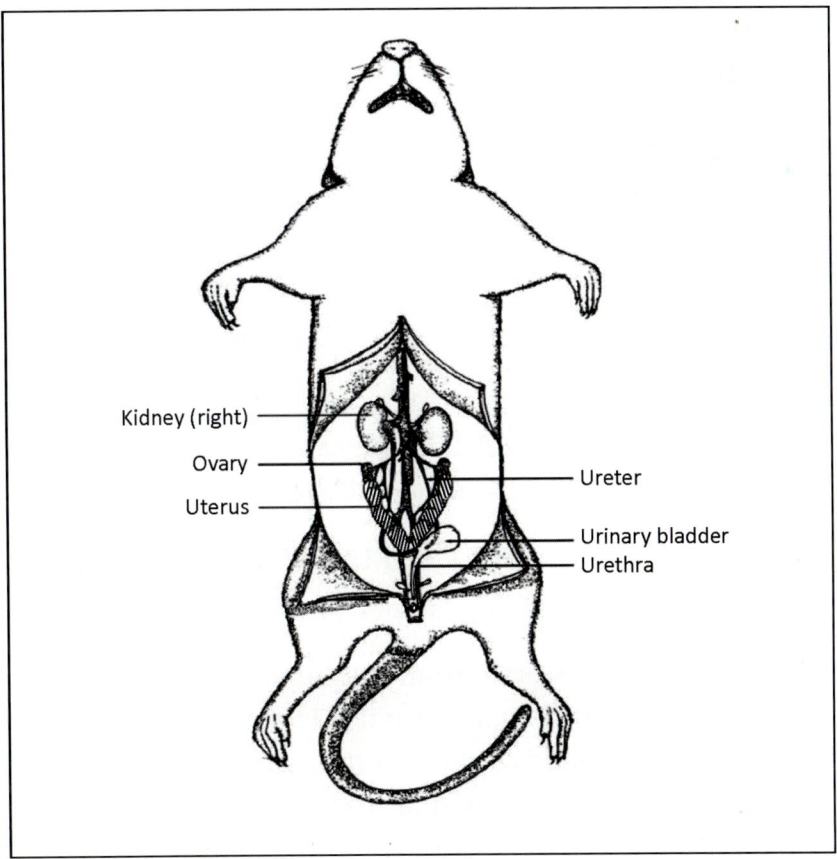

Fig. 3.22: Rat Uterus.

while other can be used later if needed. One end of the uterine horn is tied with lower end of aeration tube. The preparation is carefully transferred to organ tube filled with De-Jalon solution, in the organ bath. Other end of the tissue is then tied to the isotonic frontal writing lever. 1 g tension is applied on the lever for balancing. The tissue is allowed to equilibrate for 1 hour at 37°C.

Therapeutic relevance

Rat uterus is the most sensitive preparation for adrenaline. Rat uterus is mainly employed for studying the effects of oxytocin, adrenaline and serotonin.

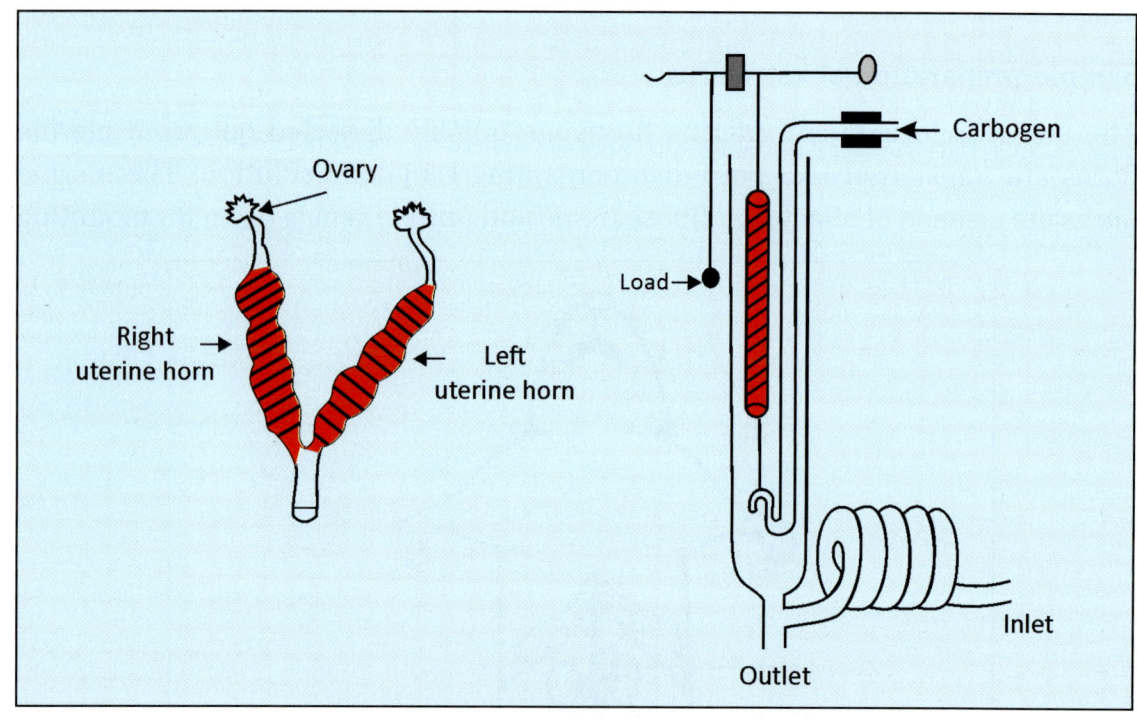

Fig. 3.23: Isolation and mounting of rat uterus.

RAT ANOCOCCYGEUS MUSCLE

Protocol for separation of tissue

The two anococcygeus muscles arise from the upper coccygeal vertebra close to one another in the midline of the pelvic cavity. The muscles pass caudally, lying first behind and then to one side of the colon, finally joining together to form a ventral bar in front of the colon a few mm from the anus. The muscle is paired, thin, consists of smooth muscle only and the muscle cells are organized in parallel bundles.

A healthy male rat weighing 200-250 g is sacrificed following all ethical norms. The abdomen is cut open in mid-line, pelvis is split and urinary bladder and urethra are gently removed without damaging the ventral band of muscles lying ventral to the colon. The colon is then cut through at the pelvic brim, the pelvic portion pulled forward and the delicate connective tissue behind cleared until the anococcygeus muscles visualised (Gillespie, 1972). The rat anococcygeus muscles are about 3 cm long, 150-300 μm thick and 0.5 cm broad at its broadest region.

Sample preparations rat annococcygeus muscle

After tracing the muscles, the threads are tied on both ends of the muscle and the individual muscle along with thread is isolated, and subsequently mounted in an organ bath containing Krebs's solution at 36°C bubbled continuously with 95% O_2 + 5% CO_2.

The preparation is allowed to stabilize for 30 min after which responses are recorded.

In some instances, anococcygeus muscles can be separated keeping the extrinsic nerve intact. The extrinsic nerves enter the deep surface of each muscle just short of the ventral band (Ghosh, 2015).

Therapeutic relevance

This smooth muscle has a dense adrenergic innervation and contracts to noradrenaline, acetylcholine, 5-hydroxytryptamine and at high concentrations to isoprenaline. No contraction is observed for histamine.

The anococcygeus muscle also contracts to field stimulation or stimulation of extrinsic nerves. The preparation can be used to assess the pre- and post-synaptic α-adrenoceptor blocking activity of drugs (Doggrell 1980).

The inhibitory response to nerve stimulation is not mimicked by acetylcholine, isoprenaline or ATP, nor blocked by atropine, phentolamine, phenoxybenzamine, propranolol, hexamethonium or lysergic acid diethylamide (Gillespie JS, 1972).

FROG RECTUS ABDOMINIS

Frog rectus abdominus muscle is a voluntary skeletal muscle producing slow contraction in response to acetylcholine (ACh). Isolated frog rectus preparation is a simple isolated tissue preparation widely used for the study of nicotinic receptors mediated effects of Ach. Since frog rectus is a skeletal muscle, nicotinic mechanism operates at neuromuscular junction. Cholinergic drugs stimulate these nicotinic receptors and produce contraction of skeletal muscle. The response of these drugs on nicotine receptors is blocked by neuromuscular blocking drug (d-tubocurarine).

Protocol for isolation of tissue

A frog is sacrificed following all ethical norms. The frog kept on the frog dissection board facing abdomen upwards. A midline incision is given, the skin of the anterior abdominal wall is cut by a midline incision which is extended laterally onto the

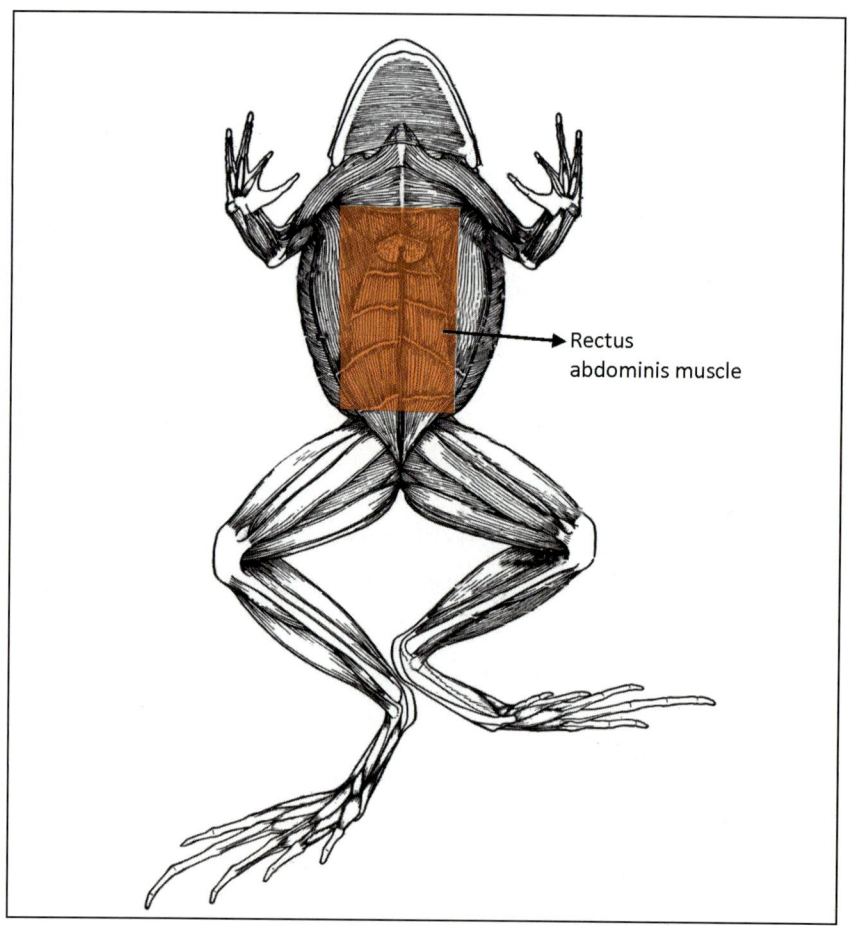

Rectus abdominis muscle

Fig. 3.24: Ventral view of rectus abdominis muscle of frog.

anterior aspects of the limbs. This exposes the flat whitish muscle of the anterior abdominal wall from their pubic origin to their sternal insertion.

Frog rectus abdominis muscle preparation

After exposing the abdominal whitish muscle, cuts are placed separately on each rectus abdominis from pelvic girdle up to the pectoral girdle. The two recti are removed and placed in Frog's Ringer solution in a shallow dish. They are carefully cleaned and one of them is trimmed to the desired size and mounted in an organ bath containing Frog Ringer solution at room temperature. The physiological salt solution is continuously bubbled with carbogen (95% oxygen and 5% carbondioxide). The muscle is allowed to equilibrate for 30 minutes before recording the drug responses.

Therapeutic relevance

Frog rectus abdominis is a valuable preparation for studying effects of agonists (e.g. ACh) and antagonists (e.g. d-tubocurarine) acting on nicotinic cholinergic receptors at neuromuscular junction.

LEECH DORSAL MUSCLE

The isolated dorsal muscle of the leech (*Hirudo medicinalis*) is employed for qualitative and quantitative bioassay of acetylcholine and nicotinic agents, to which it responds with a contracture. The sensory responses to stretch in these receptors are different from those of other more well-known muscle receptors such as vertebrate spindles or crustacean stretch receptors. The leech receptors provide the sensory innervation for the tubular muscle layers of the body wall, and they respond to stretch of the muscle with hyperpolarizing potentials that are conducted passively to the CNS (Blackshaw, 1993).

Protocol for separation of tissue

Leech is pined from both ends on a board. A longitudinal cut is given along two pale lateral line from mouth to tail of leech. All internal organs are carefully removed. Dorsal muscle is dissected out.

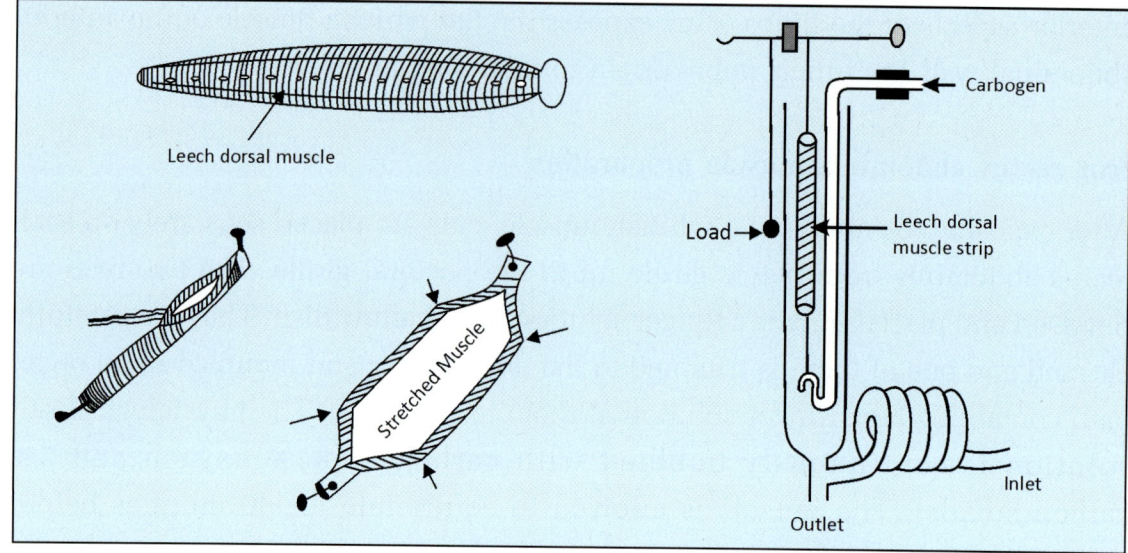

Fig. 3.25: Dorsal leech muscle and its preparation.

Leech dorsal muscle preparation

After dissecting, the dorsal muscle is separated longitudinally into two parts. Thread is tied at each end and the tissue is mounted in organ bath containing Frog-ringer or Locke's solution at room temperature.

Therapeutic relevance:

Leech dorsal muscle is a most sensitive preparation to ACh. In presence of physostigmine treatment, estimation of less than 50 picomoles concentration of ACh is possible.

References:

1. Chenoweth, M. B., and E. S. Koelle. "An isolated heart perfusion system adapted to the determination of nongaseous metabolities; with sample data upon the isolated monkey heart." The Journal of laboratory and clinical medicine 31 (1946): 600.

2. Dhalla, N. S., J. C. Yates, and V. Proveda. "Calcium-linked changes in myocardial metabolism in the isolated perfused rat heart." Canadian journal of physiology and pharmacology 55.4 (1977): 925-933.

3. Gaddum, J.H.1953, Pharmacology 4th edition pp 15.Oxford Medical Publication. Cited from Perry, W.L.M (1968). Pharmacological experiments on isolated preparations.:120.

4. Gergely, J. "Some aspects of the role of the sarcoplasmic reticulum and the tropomyosintroponin system in the control of muscle contraction by calcium ions." Circulation research 35.3 (1974): III-74.'

5. Langer, G. A. "Ionic basis of myocardial contractility." Annual review of medicine 28.1 (1977): 13-20.

6. Langer, G. A., J. S. Frank, and L. M. Nudd. "Correlation of calcium exchange, structure, and function in myocardial tissue culture." American Journal of Physiology-Heart and Circulatory Physiology 237.2 (1979): H239-H246.

7. Morad, Martin, and James Maylie. "Calcium and cardiac electrophysiology: Some experimental considerations." Chest 78.1 (1980): 166-173.

8. Neely, J.R.,H. E. Morgan,1968.Regulation of cardiac metabolism, Penn. Med. 71:57-61.

9. Neely, J. R., Liebermeister, H. Battersby, E.J., Morgan, H.E., Effect of pressure development on oxygen consumption by isolated rat heart. Am J. Physiol. 1967, 212, 804-814.

10. Philipson, Kenneth D., and Glenn A. Langer. "Sarcolemmal-bound calcium and contractility in the mammalian myocardium." Journal of molecular and cellular cardiology 11.9 (1979): 857-875.

11. Reuter, H., and N. Seitz. "The dependence of calcium efflux from cardiac muscle on temperature and external ion composition." The Journal of Physiology 195.2 (1968): 451-470.

12. Reuter, Harald. "Brief Reviews Exchange of Calcium Ions in the Mammalian Myocardium: Mechanisms and Physiological Significance." Circulation Research 34.5 (1974): 599-605.

13. Shen, Anthony C., and Robert B. Jennings. "Myocardial calcium and magnesium in acute ischemic injury." The American journal of pathology 67.3 (1972): 417.

14. Munro, A.F. Effect of autonomic drugs on the responses of isolated preparations from the guinea-pig intestine to electrical stimulation. Journal of Physiology. 1953,120,41-52.

15. Castillo, J.C. The tracheal chain; the anaphylactic guinea pig trachea and its response to antihistamine and bronchodilator drugs. J Pharmacol Exp Ther, 1948, 94, 412-415.

16. Ferre, J.P. and Ruckebusch Y. Myoelectric activity and propulsion in the large intestine of fed and fasted rats. Journal of Physiology. 1985, 362, 93-106.

17. Gillespie, J. S. The rat anococcygeus muscle and its response to nerve stimulation and to some drugs. Br. J. Pharmac.,1972,45, 404–416.

18. Ghosh MN. Editor. Fundamentals of Experimental Pharmacology. 6th Edition. Hilton and company, Kolkata; 2015, 97-106.

19. Doggrell, S.A.The assessment of pre- and postsynaptic α-adrenoceptor blocking activity of drugs using the rat anococcygeus muscle. Journal of Pharmacological Method.1980. 3, 323-331.

20. Blackshaw, S.E. Stretch receptors and body wall muscle in leeches. Camp. Eiochem. Physiol.1993,105A(4), 643-652.

4 SCREENING METHODS FOR HEPATOPROTECTIVE ACTIVITY

INTRODUCTION:

Liver is often referred as 'chemical factory' of the body, because it involves in regulation, synthesis, storage and secretion of many proteins, hormones, nutrients also in purification of toxins and unnecessary substances from the body. The risk associated with liver intoxication has recently increased by the higher exposure to environmental toxins, industrial pollutants and frequent use of chemotherapeutics along with unhealthy life-style. There are some commonly reported diseases that are associated with dysfunctioning of liver like Cirrhosis, Necrosis, Hepatitis, Hepatic failure, disorders due to impaired metabolism, Chemical(s) or drug induced hepatotoxicity.

Hepatotoxicity:

Hepatotoxicity can be produced by drugs and chemicals so hepatoprotective effect can be studied against drugs and chemicals induced hepatotoxicity in rats for e.g. alcohol, carbon- tetrachloride, galactosamine, paracetamol, antibiotics, aflatoxins and plant toxins.

Intrinsic hepatotoxins:

They are predictable hepatotoxins; they are recognized when there is a high incidence of hepatic injury. Here, consistent latent period is seen between exposure to hepatotoxins and development of hepatic injury appeared which is dose related. Intrinsic hepatotoxins are either direct acting or its metabolites or anti-metabolites (indirectly acting) which interfere with the normal metabolic pathways.

Host idiosyncrasy:

They are not predictable hepatotoxins but produces hepatic injury in only small portion. In several cases auto-antibodies against normal cellular constituents are detected. Such hepatic injury is not dose related hence it is difficult to reproduce in experimental animals.

Table 4.1: Types of Toxicity

Type of toxicity	Histological lesions	Mechanism	Example
A. Intrinsic toxicity:			
• Direct hepatotoxins	Steatosis, Necrosis	Membrane injury destruction of structural basis of cell metabolism.	Carbon tetrachloride, chloroform
• Indirect Hepatotoxins	Steatosis, Necrosis	Interfere with specific metabolic pathway leads to structural injury.	Thio-acetamide, Paracetamol, ethanol, Methotrexate, Azathioprine
• Cholestatic	Bile duct injury	Interfere with hepatic excretory pathway	Rifampicine, Steroids.
B. Host idiosyncrasy:			
• Hypersensitivity	Necrosis, Cholestasis	Drug allergy	Sulphonamide, halothane
• Metabolic abnormality	Necrosis, Cholestasis	Drug allergy	Isoniazid

EVALUATION OF HEPATOPROTECTIVE ACTIVITY:

There are many chemicals which are known hepatotoxic and used to simulate ideal liver disorders. Liver injury caused by carbon tetra-chloride, ethanol, and acetaminophen is characterized by varying degrees of cellular degeneration and cell-death, using such chemicals, liver damage is produced in experimental animals and hepatoprotective activity is measured by evaluating enzyme activities, survival ratio, and histo-archetectural studies.

Screening methods are classified as:

In-Vivo methods
In-Vitro methods

IN-VIVO methods:

Carbon tetra-chloride induced liver fibrosis in rats:

Principle:

Carbon tetrachloride is widely used for experimental induction of liver damage. Long term administration of carbon tetra-chloride to rats induces severe disturbances of hepatic function along with histologically notable liver fibrosis. After administration it undergoes metabolic reactions where it get converted into 'trichloromethyl free radical' by cytochrome P_{450} in liver microsomes, and further due to its increased concentration it leads to 'lipid peroxidation' of the membrane causes liver damage (fibrosis).

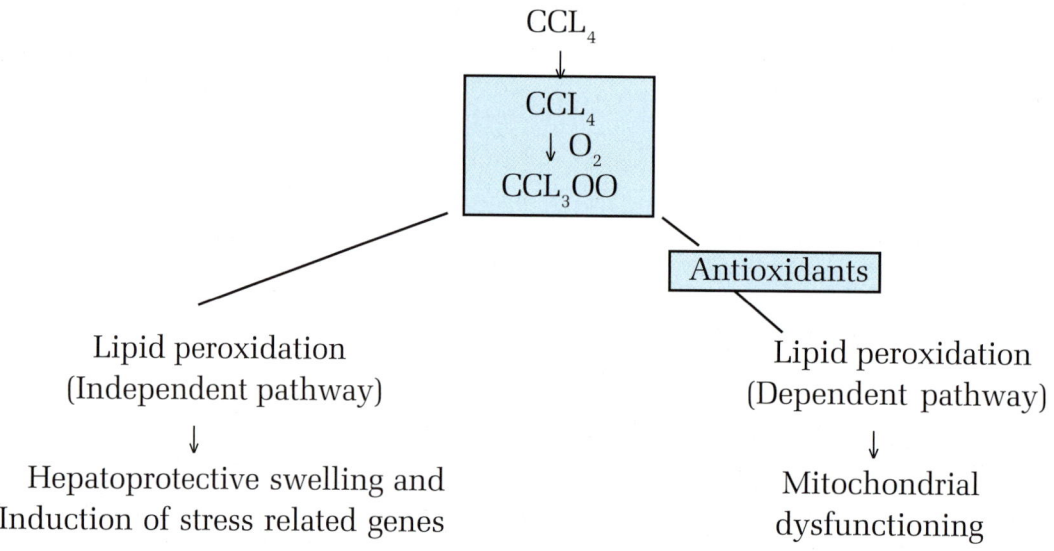

Fig. 4.1: Mechanism of hepatotoxicity induced by Carbontetra chloride.

Procedure:

Male Sprague Dawley rats (150-200 gm) are divided into 6 groups of 6 animals each.

a. Group 1 (Vehicle control)
b. Group 2 (Disease control)
c. Group 3 (Test control)
d. Group 4 (Standard control)

The test drug is administered after 6 hrs of CCL_4 treatment, 24 hrs after CCL_4 administration blood samples are withdrawn by different techniques such as (inner canthus, intravenous or by cardiac puncture) and then collected in heparinised tubes which are centrifuged at 3000 rpm for 10 min to obtain serum.

Collected blood samples are used to determine Superoxide dismutase (SOD) and to test levels of aspartate aminotransferase (AST) and alanine aminotransferase (ALT). Also the liver of each rat is promptly removed for determination of tissue SOD levels. The histological studies of hepatic tissue are performed using haematoxylin and liver slices are studied under electron microscope.

Paracetamol induced hepatotoxicity in mice:

Principle:

After administration paracetamol is metabolised by CYP_{2E1} in the liver which gives N-acetyl-P-benzoquinone molecule (NAPQI) which is again metabolised by glutathione. But when the amount of NAPQI formed is more and existing glutathione is insufficient to neutralize it, NAPQI starts binding to mitochondrial proteins and NAPQI-proteins adducts lead to necrosis of hepatocytes due to increased oxidative stress due to the free radical (NAPQI).

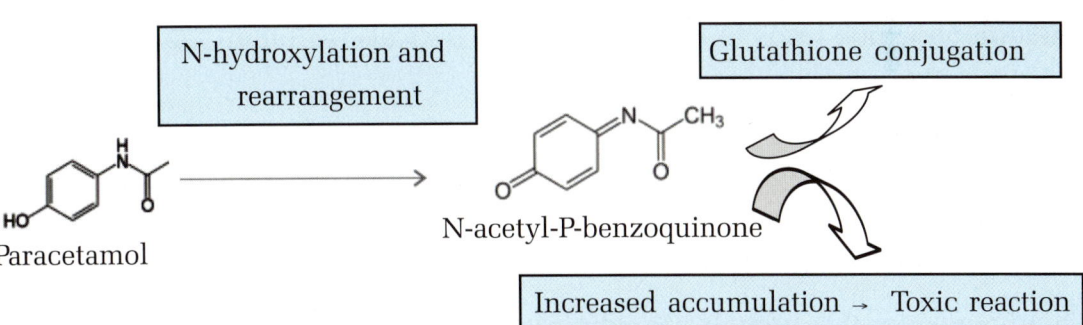

Fig. 4.2: Mechanism of hepatotoxicity induced by paracetamol.

Procedure:

The mice / rats are divided into 4 groups of 6 animals each.

a. Group A (Vehicle control)

b. Group B (Untreated control)

c. Group C (Standard control)

d. Group D (Test control)

In this model animals are treated for 7 days with the test drug and on the 7th day paracetamol (mice: 300mg/Kg, rats: 1-2g/Kg) suspension is administered orally to all the groups of rats except those in Group A. On the 8th day of the study rats are fasted overnight and sacrificed under anaesthesia.

Blood is collected and serum separated for the determination of hepatic functional parameters such as aspartate aminotransferase (AST), alanine aminotransferase (ALT), alkaline phosphatase (ALP), bilirubin are determined, and in histological studies on liver tissues collected in 10% neutral buffered formalin, slices are prepared using haematoxylin and eosin stains and observed under electron microscopy for alterations in the hepatic tissue.

Allyl alcohol induced liver necrosis in rats:
Principle:
Allyl alcohol (Prop-2-en-1-ol) is also been reported for its hepatotoxic effect in experimental animals. Hepatotoxicity of Allyl alcohol is explained on the basis of its conversion into its oxidized product, acrolein by hepatic dehydrogenase which manifest in necrosis in periportal regions of the liver lobule. Acrolein acts as high affinity substrate for the glutathione-S-transeferase, causing depletion of glutathione which leads to formation of free radicals (acrolein) known to damage hepatic cells.

Procedure:
On the first day rats are fasted, and the test compounds are administered either by orally or intraperitoneally.

One hour later, the animals are administered orally with Allyl alcohol in water and the test drug is administered after 24 hours after the Allyl alcohol administration.

After 48 hours of Allyl alcohol administration the animals are sacrificed, the liver is removed; focal necrosis is observed under the electron microscopy for the development of white/green/yellowish hemorrhagic areas in liver tissue.

The diameter of the necrotic areas is determined using ocular micrometer and the mean of the necrosis index is calculated by student's t-test so the protective effect is expressed as percentage decrease of necrosis index of the test vs. control.

Galactosamine induced liver necrosis:

Principle:

The toxic effect of galactosamine is due to insufficiency of UDP-glucose and UDP-galactose with loss of intracellular calcium homeostasis. These changes affect cell membrane, cell organelles, production of proteins and nucleic acid. Furthermore, Galactosamine is also known to interfere with the energy metabolism of hepatocytes. It interferes with enzymes involved in the transport of substrate to the mitochondria (cytochrome c oxidase) and alters the composition of phospholipids of the membrane significantly.

Procedure:

Animals are divided into two groups i.e. control and test, control group is administered with galactosamine alone while test group is administered with galactosamine and test drug.

Galactosamine is administered intraperitoneally (400 mg/kg) on 7th day after 24 hours of administration of test drug, the test drug is administered along with food or by oral route. Rats are then sacrificed after 24 hours of galactosamine injection and liver tissue is subjected for biochemical (ALT, AST, bilirubin, APT) and histological studies.

There are other *in-vivo* methods which are followed commonly, are outlined in the following table,

Table 4.2:

Chemical	Principle
Chemical induced hepatotoxicity: Thio-acetamide (Carcinogen) Induction period - 96 hours	• Liver fibrosis and cirrhosis due to oxidative stress • Formation of toxic metabolite Thio-acetamide-S-oxide which interferes with the movement of RNA from the nucleus to the cytoplasm and cause membrane injury • Damage to lipid macromolecules due to increased number of free radicals

Chemical	Principle
Azathioprine (Immunosuppressive agent) Induction period - 24 hours	• Free radicals generation leads to depletion of GSH and then mitochondrial injury. • ATP depletion • Cell death by necrosis
Isonicotinic acid hydrazide, Rifampicin, Ethambutal (Antitubercular agents) Induction period - 15 – 21 days	• Its principle metabolite undergoes dehydration to form acetyl diazine, a toxic onium ion, acetyl radical and ketene. • These metabolites bind with hepatic macromolecules causing liver injury.
Cisplatin (anticancer agent) Induction period - 24 hours	• When enters into the cell then its chloride ligands are exchanged by forming aquatic species which then react with nucleophilic sites in the cellular macromolecules (DNA) • Defects in mitochondria due to oxidative damage
Doxorubicin (anticancer agent) Induction period - 2 days	• It undergoes single electron reduction to form doxsemiquinone free radicals. • Doxsemiquinone reduces oxygen to superoxide anions and depletes antioxidant enzyme status.
Cyclosporine- A (Immunosuppressive agent) Induction period - 10 days	• Depletion of glutathione, catalase, glutathione peroxidase, superoxide dismutase
Heavy metals induced hepatotoxicity:	
Arsenic (Induction period – 24 weeks)	• Lipid peroxidation due to oxidative stress

Chemical	Principle
	• Disruption of endogenous antioxidant defence system • Increased production of inflammatory prostaglandins, cytokines and nitric oxide • Reaction of NO and superoxide anion, causes formation of peroxynitrite radicals leads to cell damage by oxidation, nitration of cellular macromolecules.
Cadmium (Induction period – 24 hours)	• Longer retention in liver • Free radicals attack the cell membrane • Destabilize, disintegrate causes lipid peroxidation
Other:	
Aflatoxin B1 (potent carcinogen produced by Aspergillus flavus)	• Metabolized to AFB1-exo-8, 9-epoxide by CYP3A4, binds with DNA guanines to form adduct leads to hepatic damage
Gamma radiation	• Hepatic cytotoxity, metabolic and morphological changes • Impairs functions of DNA, RNA, proteins, Cell membranes
Xenobiotics	• Impairment in phase II reaction causes accumulation of toxic metabolites in liver • Induction of increased intracellular calcium leads to cell death • Reduction by CYP 450 generates free radicals leads to lipid peroxidation

IN-VITRO methods:

Cytotoxicity study: Cytotoxicity is the direct toxic effect of the agents on the cells. Test drug should be devoid of any cytotoxic property. For any hepatoprotective activity drug need to be tested for its cytotoxic property. While studying *in-vitro* cytotoxicity it is essential to determine maximal effective dose, minimal effective dose and minimum cytotoxic dose range. Such exercise may help to determine the maximum hepatoprotective activity and can be studied by methods described below:

Table 4.3:

Type and nature of assay	Principle	Advantages/ Disadvantages
Cell/colony counts	Ability of hematopoietic progenitors to proliferate and differentiate into colonies.	Cumbersome, tedious, sensitive
Dye Binding (SRB assay)	A bright pink amino xanthenes dye binds to basic amino residues of proteins, colour intensity measured by using spectrophotometer.	Simple, reliable, rapid, sensitive, quantitative
Metabolic impairment (MTT assay)	Decay of Enzymatic activity, or metabolic degradation following toxic insult.	More complex, more accurate
Membrane integrity (Neutral red assay)	It is a dye that accumulates in the lysosomes of the living cells. Dead and severely traumatised cells do not accumulate and retain neutral red.	Less accurate

HepG$_2$ cell cytotoxicity study:

It is a reproducible microplate screening assay and it can be used when a large number of samples are to be analysed. Toxicity induction to the cells is done by any of the following:

a. D-galactosamine hydrochloride.
b. Tert-butyl hydroperoxide.
c. Bromobenzene.

Procedure:

HepG$_2$ are routinely grown and subcultured in monolayers. DMEM (Dulbecco's Modified Eagle's Medium) is supplemented with 10% (v/v) foetal calf serum is used as media.

Since the effect of toxins is more on matured cells, and therefore such cells are preferred for the *in-vitro* hepatoprotective studies. The negative control group cells are grown in medium alone and test groups are grown in medium with known hepatotoxins and test drug at different concentrations.

Finally cytotoxicity can be measured by viability studies of the cells. Similar viability study can be performed by applying following *in-vitro* methods:

a. MTT (3-(4,5-dimethylthiazol-2-yl)-2, 5-diphenyltetrazolium bromide assay
b. SRB (sulforhodamine B) assay
c. Tryptan blue exclusion method

Model for Anti- Hepatitis B virus:

Here, HBV DNA-transfected hepatoblastoma cell- line (2.2.15) is used because of following characteristic features:

a. It produces replicative HBV DNA intermediates
b. Produces more matured virions

The cells are first infected with HBV which is subsequently used for screening anti-Hepatitis B virus drugs.

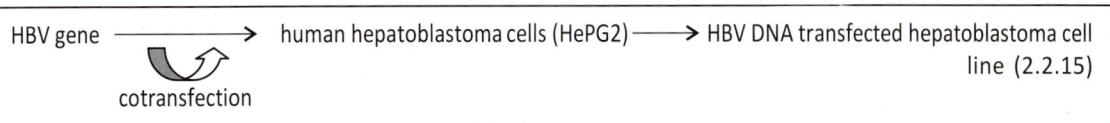

Fig. 4.3: Transfection of (HePG2) cells by HBV-DNA) Line.

Procedure:

HBV DNA- transfected hepatoblastoma cells are grown in six-well flat bottom plates. Media used is Dulbecco's modified eagle's medium, 10% FCS, 0.2 mmol/L glutamine.

Cells were incubated for 10 days in the above medium supplemented with individual antiviral drugs. The drug containing medium is added on the day one and changed every 3rd day. On the 10th day, medium and cells are harvested and analyzed.

In each experiment, 2.2.15 cells without treatment are taken as positive control. Hep G_2 cells are used as negative controls, and at last analysis has to be performed to check the viability of cells by Tryptan blue exclusion method.

Freshly isolated primary hepatocytes model:
Primary hepatocytes are used to predict the hepatoprotective nature of the drug as they provide the 'Physiological level of enzymes' and 'Intact plasma membrane' give a better correlation between *in-vivo and in-vitro* correlation. The major drawback with this method is that cells remain viable only for short period (few days).

Procedure:
The toxicity in the cells can be induced by various hepatotoxic agents like paracetamol and CCL_4. Rats are anesthetized using Phenobarbital sodium. Then heparin is injected into the femoral vein followed by perfusion with calcium free HEPES (4-(2-hydroxyethyl 1) -1-piperazineethane-sulfonic acid) buffer 20 min (37°C).

After the perfusion the lobes are removed and transferred into sterile petridish containing HEPES buffer and dispersed gently.

It is again transferred into sterile conical flask and the crude cell suspension is stirred with the help of magnetic stirrer for 5 min to release hepatocytes into the solution.

Cell viability is determined by the Tryptan blue exclusion method and isolated hepatocytes are cultured in Ham's F12 medium, supplemented with 10% newborn calf serum, antibiotics, $10^{-6}M$ dextromethasone and $10^{-8}M$ bovine insulin, then the cell suspension is incubated at 37°C for 30 min in a humidified incubator under 5% CO_2.

After 24 hours of incubation the hepatocytes are exposed to fresh medium containing paracetamol. After 1-2 hours of exposure, test drug is added and the enzyme level of AST, ALT, ALP, bilirubin and total protein is measured in the medium after 2 hours.

Acetaminophen induced hepatotoxicity in HepaRG cells:

HepaRG cells are subjected for acetaminophen overdose which results into, Glutathione depletion, protein addict formation, peroxynitrite formation, reactive oxygen species formation, mitochondrial dysfunction, and LDH release.

For acetaminophen treatment, HepaRG cells are washed with PBS (Phosphate buffered saline) and treated with acetaminophen.

Treated cells are then allowed for measuring different parameters, once the hepatotoxic condition is confirmed then the suitable concentration of test drug added and different biomarker's like AST, ALP, ALT, bilirubin are measured.

References:

1. Delgado-Montemayor, Cecilia, et al. "Models of hepatoprotective activity assessment." Medicina universitaria17.69 (2015): 222-228.

2. Farghali, H., et al. "In vitro and in vivo experimental hepatotoxic models in liver research: applications to the assessment of potential hepatoprotective drugs." Physiological research 65 (2016).

3. Ingawale, Deepa K., Satish K. Mandlik, and Suresh R. Naik. "Models of hepatotoxicity and the underlying cellular, biochemical and immunological mechanism (s): a critical discussion." Environmental toxicology and pharmacology 37.1 (2014): 118-133.

4. Koblihová, Eva, et al. "Acute liver failure induced by thioacetamide: Selection of optimal dosage in Wistar and Lewis rats." Physiological Research 63.4 (2014): 491.

5. Lim, Hwa-Kyung, et al. "Effects of acetylbergenin against D-galactosamine-induced hepatotoxicity in rats." Pharmacological Research 42.5 (2000): 471-474.

6. McGill, Mitchell R., et al. "Acetaminophen-induced liver injury in rats and mice: comparison of protein adducts, mitochondrial dysfunction, and oxidative stress in the mechanism of toxicity." Toxicology and applied pharmacology 264.3 (2012): 387-394.

7. Ohno, Yasuo, et al. "Mechanism of allyl alcohol toxicity and protective effects of low-molecular-weight thiols studies with isolated rat hepatocytes." Toxicology and applied pharmacology 78.2 (1985): 169-179.

5 METHODS FOR SCREENING ANTI-HYPERGLYCEMIC AGENTS

INTRODUCTION AND PHARMACOTHERAPY

Diabetes mellitus is a chronic metabolic disorder characterized by hyperglycemia associated with carbohydrate, fat and protein metabolism caused by deficiency in insulin secretion or decreased sensitivity of the tissues to insulin action (insulin resistance).

The main cause of hyperglycaemia is uncontrolled hepatic glucose output and reduced uptake of glucose by skeletal muscle accompanied by reduced glycogen synthesis. The symptoms are glycosuria, polyuria, dehydration, thirst and increased intake of fluids (polydipsia). Insulin deficiency causes wasting due to increased breakdown and reduced synthesis of proteins. The are two main types of diabetes mellitus are:

1) **Type 1 diabetes - Insulin-dependent diabetes mellitus (IDDM)**
2) **Type 2 diabetes - Non-insulin-dependent diabetes mellitus (NIDDM)**

Insulin is essential for the treatment of type 1 diabetes. The type 2 diabetes (NIDDM) treated with various class of oral hypoglycemic agents such as Sulphonylureas, Meglitinides, Thiazolidinediones, Bigunides and α-glucosidase inhibitors. In addition to these, the new class of compounds viz., GLP-1 agonist, DPP-IV inhibitors, SGLT-2 inhibitors are used in treatment of diabetes mellitus.

ANIMAL MODELS OF DIABETES

To study the effect of experimental molecules for their efficacy in diabetes, the experimental drugs/extracts can be administered for three weeks before the induction of the disorder (prophylactic evaluation) or the treatment can be carried out for three weeks after diabetes has been induced (therapeutic evaluation). The time period can be varied depending on the experimental drugs/extracts under evaluation.

ALLOXAN INDUCED DIABETES (Szkedelski, 2001, Frode, 2008)

Alloxan (2,4,5,6-tetraoxypyrimidine) has two distinct pathological effects. It causes selective inhibition of insulin secretion that is triggered by a rise in glucose through inhibition of glucokinase (the glucose sensor of the beta cell). This causes generation of reactive oxygen species (ROS) and necrosis of beta cells, which leads to insulin dependent. Alloxan accumulates in the beta cells and causes damage to the cells. Alloxan and its reduction form, dialuric acid, establish a redox cycle with the formation of superoxide radicals. As a result of this reaction, hydrogen peroxide is formed and there is a massive increase in cytosolic calcium concentration, leading to rapid destruction of pancreatic beta cells.

The most frequently used intravenous dose of alloxan in rats is 65 mg/kg, but when it is administered intraperitoneally or subcutaneously its effective dose must be higher. For instance, an intraperitoneal dose below 150 mg/kg may be inadequate for inducing diabetes in animal species. In mice, doses vary among 100–200 mg/kg by intravenous route (i.v.).

STREPTOZOTOCIN INDUCED DIABETES (Rees and Alcolado, 2005)

Streptozotocin (STZ, 2-deoxy-2-(3-(methyl-3-nitrosoureido)-D-glucopyranose), synthesized by *Streptomycetes achromogenes*, is used for experimental induction of both insulin-dependent and non-insulin-dependent diabetes mellitus depending on the dose (IDDM and NIDDM, respectively).

Streptozotocin is a nitrosourea analogue in which the *N*-methyl-*N*-nitrosourea moiety is linked to the carbon-2 of a hexose. It is selectively accumulated in pancreatic beta cells via the low affinity glucose transporter (GLUT-2) in the plasma membrane. Its methylnitrosourea moiety, especially at the O-6 position of guanine, alkylates the DNA thus leading to toxicity. This alkylation causes damage and subsequently leads to the fragmentation of the DNA. In the attempt to repair DNA, poly (ADP-ribose) polymerase (PARP) is over stimulated. This diminishes cellular NAD^+, and subsequently ATP stores. The depletion of the cellular energy stores ultimately results in beta cell necrosis. Protein methylation also occurs and this contributes to the functional defects of the β–cells after exposure to streptozotocin.

The most commonly employed dose of STZ in adult rats is 60 mg/kg to induce insulin dependent diabetes. Higher doses are also used. STZ can also be administered intraperitoneally in a single dose < 40 mg/kg. Diabetes is considered to be induced if the blood glucose concentrations in fed animals are greater than 200–300 mg/dl, 2 days after STZ injection. A model of type 2 diabetes can be induced in rats by either i.v. (tail vein) or i.p. treatment with STZ in the first days of life. At 8–10 weeks old and thereafter, rats neonatally treated with STZ manifest mild basal hyperglycemia, an impaired response to the glucose tolerance test, and a loss of pancreatic β-cell sensitivity to glucose. STZ given in multiple low doses (40 mg/kg, i.v. for 5 days), in adult mice induces an insulin dependent diabetes

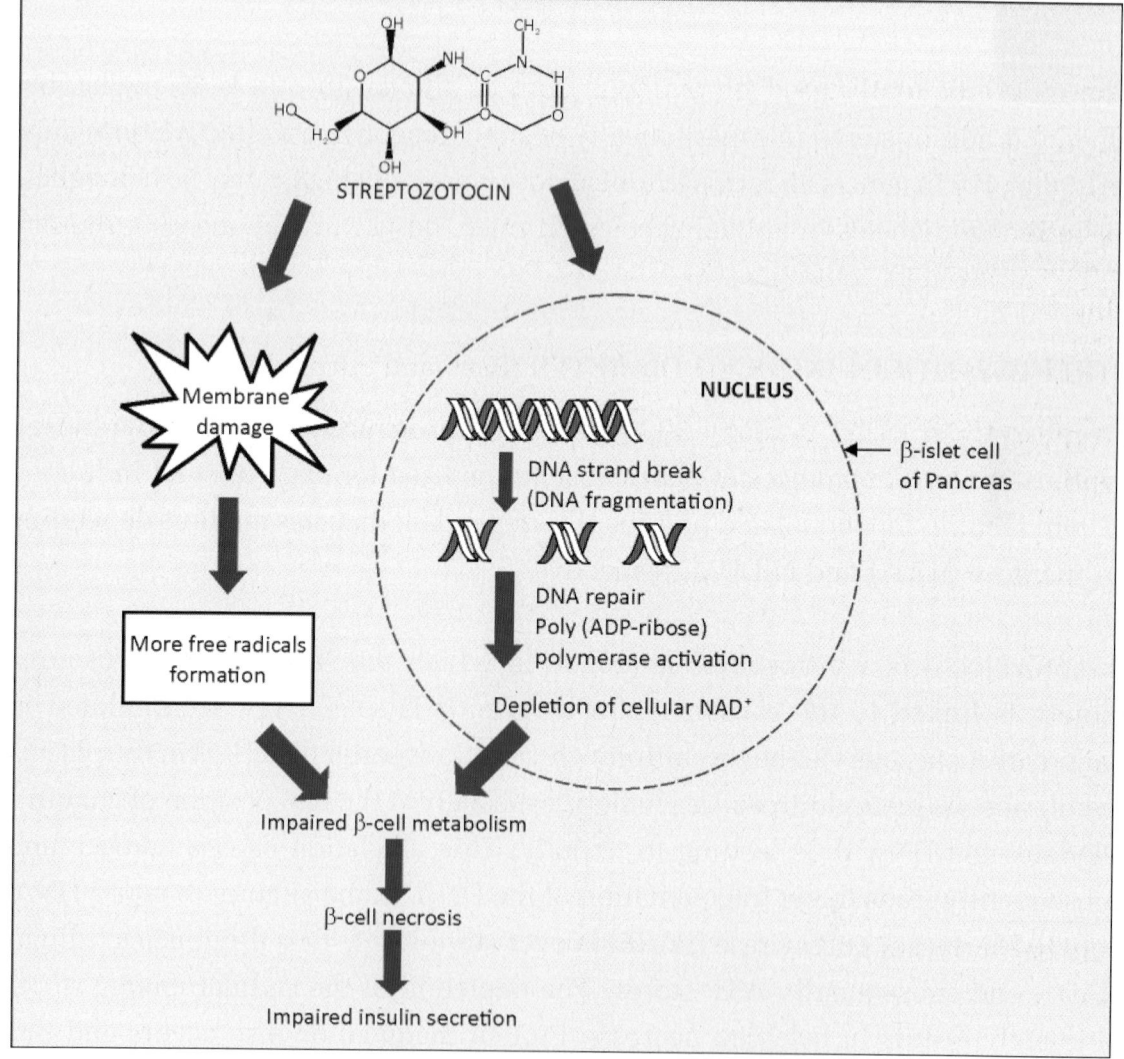

Fig. 5.1: Mechanism of action of Streptozotocin.

that is quite similar to the autoimmune forms (islet degeneration and β-cell destruction) of type 1 diabetes. On the other hand, a single dose between 60 and 100 mg/kg of STZ, administered systemically can also cause insulin dependent diabetes, but it lacks the autoimmune profile. The potential problem with STZ is that its toxic effects are not restricted to pancreatic β-cells since it may cause renal injury, oxidative stress inflammation and endothelial dysfunction.

GENETIC MODELS FOR ANTIDIABETIC TESTING (Kumar et al., 2004, Frode, 2008)

Rodents have been described to exhibit spontaneous diabetes mellitus on a hereditary basis. Such animals models give more insight into the pathogenesis of diabetes in human beings. Some of these animal models are described in following:

Table 5.1: List of Genetic models for Antidiabetic screening

Animal Model	Pathophysiologic Mechanism	Diasease Condition
RAT		
Bio-Breeding (BB) Rat	Spontneous diabetes due to auto immune destruction of the pancreatic β-cells	IDDM
WBN/Kob rat	Impaired glucose tolerance and glucosuria at 21 weeks of age	IDDM
Got-Kakizaki (GK) rat	GK rats are non-obese, insulin-resistant. 2 to 4 weeks after birth defects in glucose stimulated insulin secretion, peripheral insulin resistance, and hyper insulinemia are seen along with impaired skeletal muscle glycogen synthase activation by insulin.	NIDDM
Zuker-fatty rat	Hyper insulinemic obesity. Obesity occurs due to a simple autosomal recessive (fa) gene at an early age	NIDDM

Animal Model	Pathophysiologic Mechanism	Diasease Condition
OLETS rat	Characteristic features of OLETS rats are: (1) hyperglycemia onset is late (after 18 weeks of age), (2) a chronic course of disease, (3) mild obesity, (4) inheritance by males, (5) hyperplastic foci of pancreatic islets, and (6) renal complications nodular lesions).	NIDDM
Obese SHR rat	Spontaneously hypertensive female rat with Obesity, hyper triglyceridemia and hyper insulinemia	NIDDM
MOUSE		
KK Mouse	Moderatly obese animals showing polyphagia, polyuria with glycosuria and blood sugar levels upto 320 mg% at the age of 7 months or older	NIDDM
KK-AY Mouse	Blood glucose and circulating insulin levels as well as HbA1c levels are increased progressively from 5 weeks of age. Degranulation and glycogen infiltration of β-cells and lipogenesis by liver and adipose tissue are increased.	NIDDM
NOD Mouse	Hypoinsulinemia secondary to autoimmune destruction of pancreatic β-cells.	IDDM
Diabetes Mouse (db/db)	Autosomal recessive mutation in the leptinreceptor gene. Characterized by hyperinsulinemia, and hyperglycemia	NIDDM

Animal Model	Pathophysiologic Mechanism	Diasease Condition
	HAMSTER	
Wellesley mouse	Elevated levels of immunoreactive insulin in serum, enlarged pancreatic islets and reduced insulin responsiveness in peripheral tissues	NIDDM
Chinese Hamster	Severe polyuria, glucosuria, ketonuria, and proteinuria; pathological changes are seen in sections of pancreas, liver and kidney. The numbers of pancreatic islets are decreased and the cells of the remaining islets are abnormal.	Mild Hyperglycemia – NIDDM, Severe-IDDM

PARAMETERS TO BE EVALUATED TO STUDY THE EFFECT OF EXPERIMENTAL MOLECULES IN DIABETES

- Blood glucose and glycosylated hemoglobin (HbA1c) levels.
- Hepatic glycogen content and oral glucose tolerance test (OGTT).
- After the completion of the study, the animals are sacrificed and the homogenate of pancreas are prepared to evaluate the following parameters: MDA, GSH, SOD and catalase content in pancreas tissue homogenate.

References:

1. Szkudelski, T., The mechanism of alloxan and streptozotocin action in B cells of the rat pancreas. Physiol Res., 2001, 50(6), 537-546.

2. Kumar, S., Singh, R., Vasudeva, N., Sharma, S., Acute and chronic animal models for the evaluation of anti-diabetic agents. Cardiovasc Diabetol., 2012, 11, 9.

3. Rees, D. A., Alcolado, J. C., Animal models of diabetes mellitus. Diabet Med., 2005, 22(4), 359-70.

4. Fröde, T.S., Medeiros, Y.S., Animal models to test drugs with potential antidiabetic activity. J Ethnopharmacol., 2008, 115(2), 173-83.

METHODS FOR SCREENING ANTI-HYPERLIPIDEMIC AGENTS

INTRODUCTION AND PHARMACOTHERAPY

Hyperlipidemia is a common metabolic syndrome characterized by abnormal blood lipid profiles, indexed by increased levels of total cholesterol (TC), triglyceride (TG), low-density lipoprotein cholesterol (LDL-C) and decreased level of high-density lipoprotein cholesterol (HDL-C).

Hyperlipidemia may induce atherosclerosis, which is a major risk factor for cardiovascular and cerebrovascular disease, such as coronary heart disease, stroke, and myocardial infarction. The endogenous Cholesterol biosynthetic pathway is mainly controlled by a rate limiting enzyme, 3-hydroxy-3-methylglutaryl-CoA (HMG-CoA) reductase, which catalyzes the conversion of HMG-CoA into mevalonic acid. Thus, this enzyme is the target of the widely available drugs that reduce Cholesterol levels, known as **statins**, which inhibit HMG-CoA reductase. However, several adverse effects, including asymptomatic creatine kinase elevation in muscles and rhabdomyolysis, have been associated with statins, prompting the search for safe and effective strategies to treat hyperlipidemia. **Fibrates** have several beneficial effects on lipid metabolism, all of which appear to be secondary to the activation of the transcription factor, Peroxisome proliferator-activated receptor α (PPARα). Fibrates bind to PPARα which is expressed primarily in the liver and brown adipose tissue and to a lesser extent in kidneys, heart and skeletal muscle. The two established **bile-acid sequestrants** or resins (**cholestyramine** and **colestipol**) are most often used as second agents if statin therapy does not lower LDL-C levels sufficiently. When used with a statin, cholestyramine and colestipol usually are prescribed at submaximal doses. **Colesevelam** is a newer bile-acid sequestrant that is prepared as an anhydrous gel or suspension. The bile-acid sequestrants are highly positively charged and bind to the negatively charged bile acids. The resins-bile salt complex cannot be reabsorbed in the distal ileum, and the bound bile acids are excreted in the stool. There are two available cholesterol absorption inhibitors: **plant sterols/stanols** and **Ezetimibe**. Ezetimibe is used primarily as an adjuvant along with statins. Plant sterols/stanols are similar in molecular structure to cholesterol, but are substantially more hydrophobic. As a result they displace cholesterol from micelles, increasing loss of cholesterol in stools. Plant sterols/stanols are themselves poorly absorbed. Ezetimibe at very low concentrations reduces intestinal cholesterol absorption by about 50%. It reduces cholesterol movement from micelles into the enterocyte by inhibiting uptake through the brush border protein NPC1L1.

ANIMAL MODELS OF HYPERLIPIDEMIA

To study the effect of experimental molecules for their efficacy in hyperlipidemia, the experimental drugs/extracts can be dosed for three weeks before the induction of the disorder (prophylactic evaluation) or the treatment can be initiated for three weeks after the establishment of hyperlipidemia (therapeutic evaluation). The time period can be varied depending on the experimental drugs/extracts under evaluation.

High fat diet (HFD) / fat emulsion induced (Zhang et al, 2017)

Male Wistar/Sprague-Dawley rats weighing 180–220 g can be used for this model. Fat emulsion (consisting of 25% lard, 1% cholesterol, 1% propylthiouracil, 25% Tween-80 and 20% propylene glycol) is administered for 30 days or high fat diet comprising 68% basal diet, 10% sugar, 10% yolk powder, 10% lard and 2% cholesterol for 6 weeks is provided instead of standard pellet diet. Atorvastatin or simvastatin can be used as standard drugs to compare the activity of the experimental compounds.

Lipid and sucrose induced (Madariaya et al, 2015)

BALB/c mice should be administered modified standard diet in which 20% of the diet (by weight) is substituted with lard (46% saturated fat, 44% unsaturated fat) and sucrose-containing drinking water. To prepare the modified diet, 80 g of chow was homogenized with 20 g of lard in distilled water at 50°C in an automatic mixer and then dried it into pellets.

High fructose diet induced (Putakala et al, 2017)

Male Wistar rats weighing 140-160 g can be used for the study. Fructose diet contained 66% of fructose is provided instead of normal pellet diet for 60 days.

Composition of the high fructose diet is as follows: 66% fructose, 18% protein, 8% fat, 4% cellulose, 3% AIN-93G mineral mix and 1% AIN-93G vitamin mix. Pioglitazone can be used as standard drugs to compare the activity of the experimental compounds.

Surfactant induced (Sousa et al, 207)

Male Wistar rats weighing between 300 g and 360 g can be used for this model. Tyloxapol (Triton WR 1339) is a nonionic surfactant that has been widely used to induce acute hyperlipidemia in animal models, in order to screen lipid-lowering natural or chemical drugs and to study Cholesterol and TG metabolism. Tyloxapol (400 mg/kg,i.p.) increases plasma Cholesterol levels by promoting hepatic Cholesterol synthesis, particularly via increased HMG-CoA reductase activity. The hepatic HMG-CoA reductase activity in rats treated with tyloxapol increases by 3.59 times as compared to the negative control group. In addition, tyloxapol directly disturbs lipolytic enzymes responsible for hydrolysis of plasma lipids, such as lipoprotein lipases, thus blocking the uptake of lipids from circulation to extra-hepatic tissues, resulting in increased blood lipid concentration. Atorvastatin or Simvastatin can be used as standard drugs to compare the activity of the experimental compounds. Poloxamer 407 (P407) is a ubiquitous manmade surfactant and non-ionic detergent, that across the BBB. It has been observed that P407 induces hyperlipidemia in experimental animals after parenteral administration. Typically, cholesterol and triglycerides increase within 36 hours, of a single intraperitoneal injection of 500 mg/kg of P407. P407 facilitates hypercholesterolemia due to indirect stimulation of the activity of 3-hydroxy-3-methylglutaryl coenzyme A (HMG CoA) reductase while decreasing low density lipoprotein (LDL) receptor expression in the liver.

GENETIC MODELS

Apolipoprotein E genetically deleted (ApoE–/–) micefed with HFD (Pattersonet al., 2013)

It has been found that the fibrinolytic system is impaired in ApoE–/– mice due to increased levels of plasminogen activator inhibitor-1 (PAI-1), the main regulator of this system, leading to an increase in venous thrombosis. Apolipoprotein E (ApoE) is a class of apolipoproteins with biological functions of transporting lipoproteins, fat-soluble vitamins and cholesterol into the lymph system and then into the blood. It is mainly involved in cardiovascular disease. It has been demonstrated that when ApoE–/– mice are fed a high-fat diet, there is a greater probability of developing atherosclerosis and excessive accumulations of TC and LDL-C around vascular walls are observed.

Parameters to be evaluated to study the effect of experimental molecules in hyperlipidemia

- The following serum parameters are to be evaluated: Serum lipid profile (TC, TG, HDL-C, LDL-C, VLDL-C).

- Based on the serum lipid profile, the Atherosclerosis indices can be calculated as follows: Atherosclerosis Index (A.I) = LDL-C / HDL-C, Cardiac Risk Ratio (C.R.R)=TC/HDL-C, Atherogenic Coefficient (A.C) = TC-HDL-C/HDL-C.

- After the completion of the study, the animals are sacrificed and the homogenate of liver and cardiac tissue are prepared to evaluate the following parameters:
  Hepatic and cardiac lipid content: Cholesterol and triglycerides
  Anti-oxidant effect: MDA, GSH, SOD and catalase content in hepatic tissue homogenate

- The faecal matter of the animals is to be collected on the last three days of the study and the cholesterol content in the faecal matter is estimated.

- Histopathological evaluation of liver and aorta by H & E staining can be carried out after preserving the respective tissues in 10% formalin after sacrificing the animals.

References:

1. Madariaga, Y.G,, Cárdenas, M.B., Irsula, M.T., Alfonso, O.C., Cáceres, B.A., Morgado, E.B., Assessment of four experimental models of hyperlipidemia. 2015 Apr;44(4):135-40.

2. Zhang, Y., Wang, Z., Jin, G., Yang, X., Zhou, H., Regulating dyslipidemia effect of polysaccharides from Pleurotus ostreatus on fat-emulsion-induced hyperlipidemia rats.Int J Biol Macromol. 2017 Aug;101:107-116.

3. Putakala, M., Gujjala, S., Nukala, S., Bongu, S.B.R., Chintakunta, N., Desireddy, S.. Cardioprotective effect of Phyllanthus amarus against high fructose diet induced myocardial and aortic stress in rat model. Biomedicine & Pharmacotherapy. 2017, 95, 1359-1368.

4. de Sousa, J.A., Pereira, P., Allgayer, M.D.C., Marroni, N.P., de Barros Falcão Ferraz A.B., Picada, J.N., Evaluation of DNA damage in Wistar rat tissues with hyperlipidemia induced by tyloxapol. Experimental and Molecular Pathology, 2017, 103, 51-55.

5. Patterson, K.A.,Zhang, X.,Wrobleski S.K., Hawley, A.E., Lawrence, D.A., Wakefield,T.W., Myers,D.D., Diaz, J.A.Rosuvastatin reduced deep vein thrombosis in ApoE gene deleted mice with hyperlipidemia through non-lipid lowering effects. Thrombosis Research, 2013, 131, 268-276.

INFLAMMATORY PROCESS AND RESPONSES

Inflammation has been variously defined. It is an endogenous protective reaction to tissue injury. Hence, it is a protective and normal response to any kind of noxious stimulus. The stimulus likely to alter the normal physiological processes of the host, may vary from acute transient and highly localized response to simple mechanical injury, or to the complex persistent response involving whole organism. Thus, inflammation is the body's defense mechanism to inactivate or destroy invading external agents such as chemical, biological or microbiological organism, remove them and prepare a stage for tissue repair. Therefore inflammation can be broadly defined by summing up all these indogenous processes, as a complex, vascular lymphatic and local tissue response induced in animals by using viable and nonviable irritants. The cardinal signs of inflammation are heat, pain, redness, swelling and loss of function.

CLASSIFICATION OF INFLAMMATION

The inflammation may be broadly classified into various categories such as:

- Acute inflammation

- Sub chronic inflammation

- Chronic inflammation

- Miscellaneous
  The acute inflammatory response encompasses a complex well coordinated cascade events involving a large number of pharmacological, physiological, chemical and molecular changes.

  Inflammatory responses occur in three distinct phases and each one of them is apparently mediated by different mechanisms.

1. An acute transient phase characterized by local vasodilation and increased capillary permeability.

2. Delayed subacute phase, most prominently characterized by infiltration of leukocytes and phagocytes.

3. A chronic proliferative phase, in which tissue degeneration, fibrosis and development of scar tissue formation.

1) Reaction/Responses during inflammation

The various cellular, vascular, physiological and pathological changes occurring during inflammation have helped to simulate screening models both *in-vivo* and *in-vitro*, and given impetus to develop better and more effective drugs.

EXPERIMENTAL METHODS FOR EVALUATION OF ANTI-INFLAMMATORY ACTIVITY

Wide variety of animal models of inflammation are experimentally simulated by considering various responses of the living tissue injury, systemic reactions and

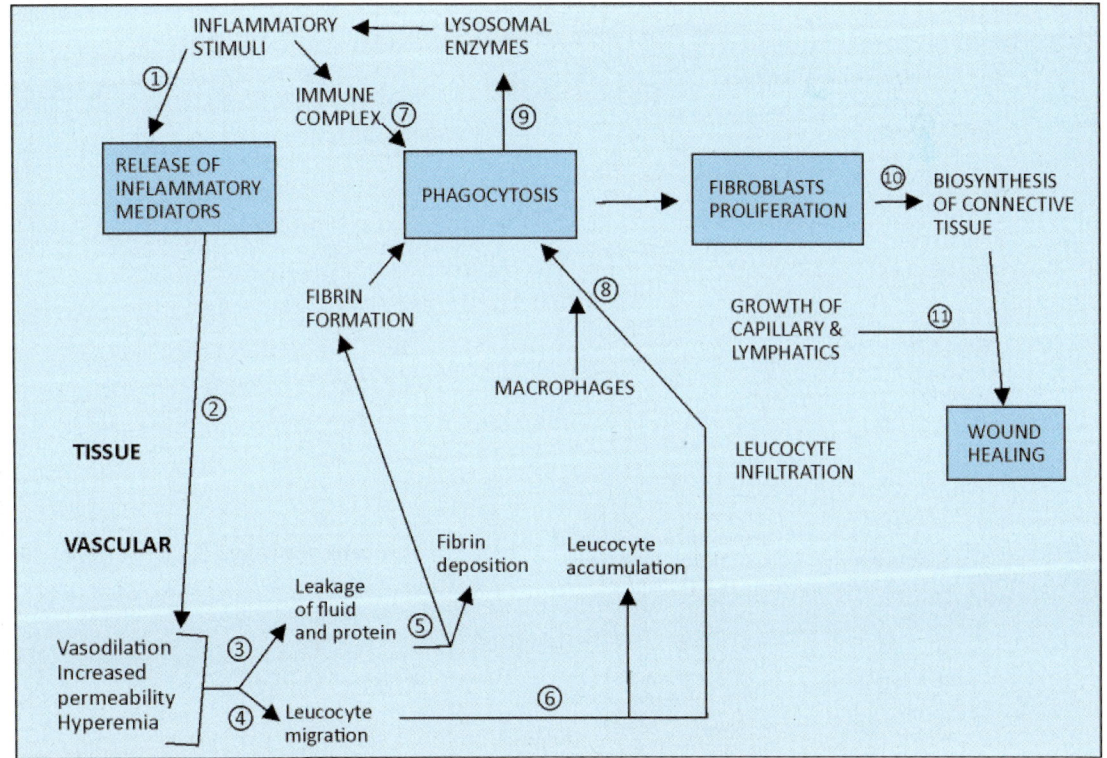

Fig. 7.1: The figure illustrate various events-physiological, pharmacological, chemical and molecular alterations during the different phases of inflammation.

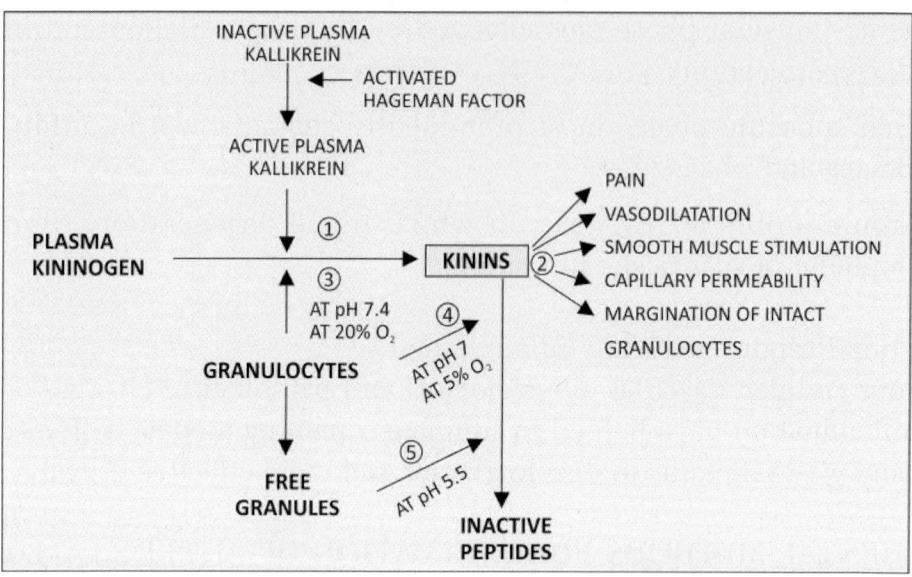

Fig. 7.2: The figure depicts the participation of kallikrein and kinins in inflammatory process.

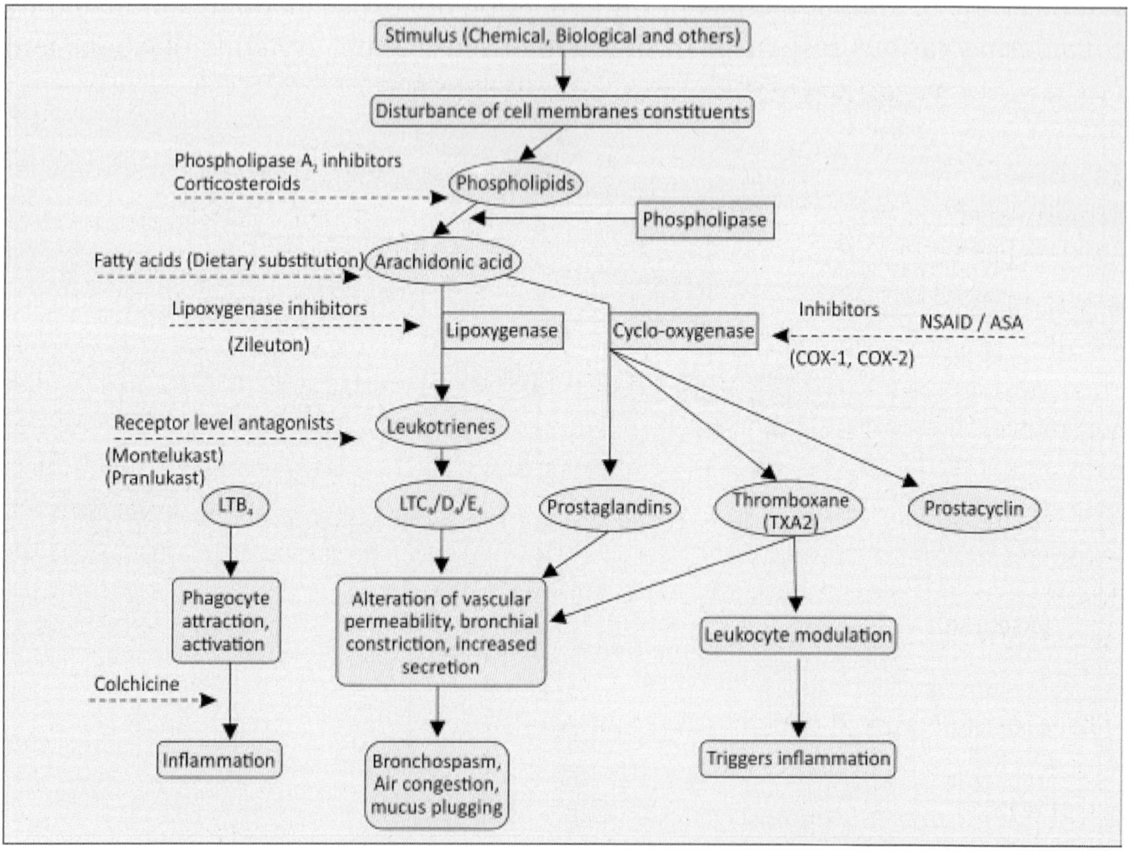

Fig. 7.3: Participation of Arachidonic acid derived mediators in inflammatory process and underlying mechanisms of Anti-inflammatory drugs (steroidal and non-steroidal).

large number of cellular, biochemical and molecular alterations in different connective tissues, bones, tendons, heart valves and joints. The cardinal signs of inflammation are pain, edema, redness, heat and ultimately lead to loss of function. The major critical responses/reactions of inflammation render themselves readily to measure erythema (local vasodilatation), edema (increased vascular permeability), and finally leading to formation of granular tissue.

Bioassay methods of Inflammation

Erythema assay:

Two types of erythema are commonly produced by irradiation with ultraviolet light in guinea pig and rat. In humans, erythema is produced by rubbing the skin with specific irritants such as 5% tetrahydrofurfuryl-nicotinate cream. Ultraviolet irradiation of mouse skin also leads to the formation of erythema. The erythema formation is inhibited by most of the anti-inflammatory drugs.

Prostaglandin E levels in the skin are elevated during the 24 hour period following exposure of guinea pig skin to ultraviolet radiation at 280-320 nm.

In this type of assay, generally guinea pigs Dunkin Hartly strain of either sex weighing 400-450 g are used. The dorsal part of the animals shaved with the help of electric clipper 18 hours prior to testing. Then they are chemically depilated by a commercial depilation product or by a suspension of barium sulphide. The depilation paste and fur are rinsed off, in running warm water. On the following day, half of the test drug dose is administered orally 30 minutes before UV exposure. The control animals are treated with normal saline/vehicle. The guinea pigs are placed in a leather cuff with a hole of 1.5 × 2.5 cm size punched on it, allowing the UV radiation to reach only the right (marked) area. Then animals are exposed to UV radiation. After 2 minutes of exposure, the remaining half of the test drug dose is administered. The erythema is scored in a double blinded manner, at 2 and 4 hours after exposure.

The scoring erythema system is as follows:

No erythema	-	0
Mild edema	-	2
Marked erythema	-	3
Marked erythema with edema	-	4

The total score after 2 and 4 hours indicate duration of action of drug as well as peak hour effect. ED_{50} values can also be calculated using different doses of reference drug and test compound.

Vascular Permeability:

Vascular permeability is increased during inflammation. The test is deviced to assess the inhibitory effect of a drug on vascular permeability induced by phlogistic agents. Inflammatory mediators such as histamine, prostaglandins and leukotrienes are released from mast cells and leukocytes, following administration of phlogistic agent, that induces vasodilation of arterioles and venules, and finally manifest in increased vascular permeability.

Rat/mouse are used in this experiment. Test drugs are administered by intraperitoneal/oral route. One hour later, animals are injected with acetic acid (1 ml/100 g of 0.6% v/v solution) intraperitoneally. Immediately 10 ml/kg of 10% w/v Evan's blue is administered intravenously via caudal vein. Thirty minutes later the animals are anaesthetized with ether anesthesia and sacrificed. The abdomen is cut open and exposed viscera. The animals are held by a flap of abdominal wall over a petri dish. The peritoneal fluid (exudates) is collected, filtered and final volume is made up to 10 ml with normal saline solution and centrifuged at 3000 rpm for 15 minutes. The absorbance of this supernatant is measured at 590 nm on a spectrophotometer. The decreased concentration of dye with respect to absorbance suggests decreased vascular permeability. The result of test compound is compared with that of reference drug. ED_{50} values are calculated or dose response curve - (drug dose against percent inhibition in dye concentration) can be plotted.

Oxazolone-induced ear edema in mice

The oxazolone induced ear edema model in mice represent delayed contact hypersensitivity and useful in assessing quantitative evaluation of topical and systemic anti-inflammatory activity of drug. The oxazolone-repeated challenge increases the level of the cytokines and decreases that of Th_2 cytokines in the lesioned skin. The Th_2 cytokines, especially IL-4 play a major role in the development of dermatitis in the mouse model. Briefly, the mice are divided into different groups and skin site of the right ear is sensitized by a single application of 10 μl (each 5 μl for inner and outer ear) of 0.5% oxazolone in acetone, 7 days

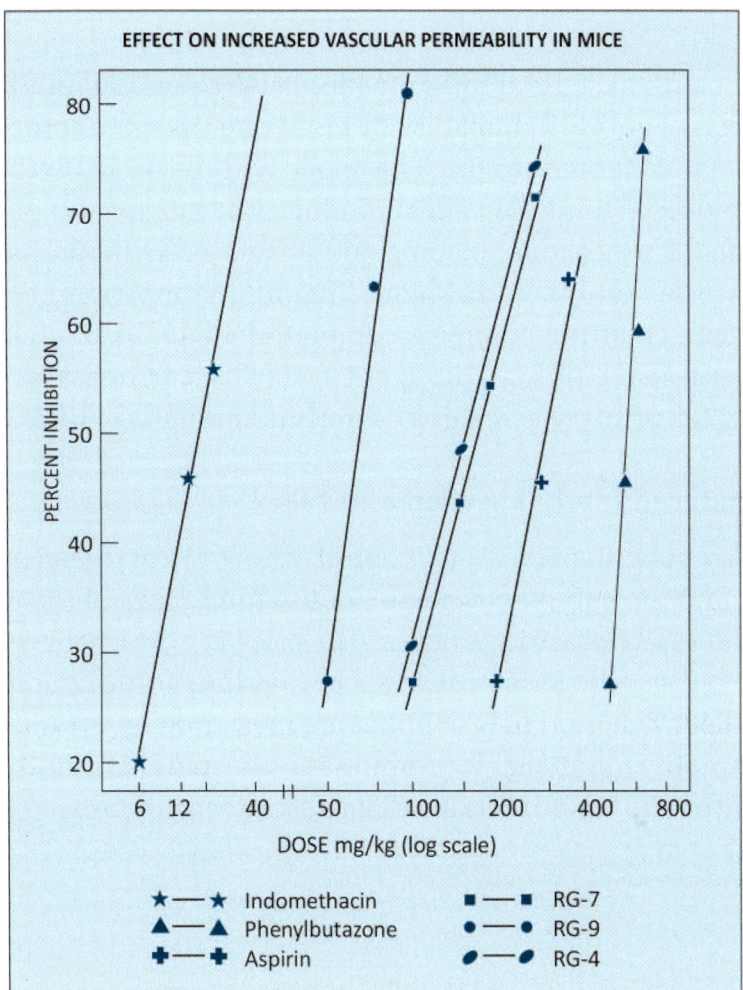

Fig. 7.4: Effect of anti-inflammatory drugs on capillary permeability in mice.

prior to first challenge (day zero) and 10 μl of 0.5% oxazolone in acetone is repeatedly applied topically to the sensitized right ear 3 times/week.

In the non-sensitized animals, only acetone is applied to the right ear. The left ear remains untreated. The maximum inflammation occurs within 24 hours after the last topical applicaion. At this time the animals are sacrificed under anesthesia, and disc of 8 mm diameter is punched from both sides. The disc is immediately weighed on a precision balance. The difference of weight between right and left ear is an indication of inflammatory reaction (edema formation). The average increase in weight is calculated for each test drug treated dose and compared with that of control group. A dose response curve can be plotted and ED_{50} values are also determined.

Edema assay

Each one of the cardinal signs of inflammation have been used in various methods for the evaluation of anti-inflammatory drugs at one time or another in the search of anti-inflammatory compounds. The most widely used method is the one involving inhibition of hind paw edema induced in rats by sub plantar injection of local irritants. The various edemogenic agents or irritants used are: dilute formalin, egg white, kaolin, carrageenan, naphthoylheparamine, brewer yeast, dextran, serotonin, creatinin complex, compound 48/80, histamine and mustard. The most widely used phlogistic agent today is carrageenan (a sulphated polysaccharide) for primary screening of anti-inflammatory drugs.

Carrageenan induced hind paw edema in rats

Rats are injected subcutaneously (0.1 ml of 1% w/v) carrageenan (prepared in normal saline) into the sub plantar region of the hind paws of the rats. Test drugs are administered orally at various doses 1 hr prior to carrageenan injection. One group of rats served as vehicle control. In such experiments the time course response can also be studied. The hind paw volumes are measured by volume displacement method using plethysmometer by immersing the paw till the level of lateral malleolus at different time intervals. The results are expressed as percentage

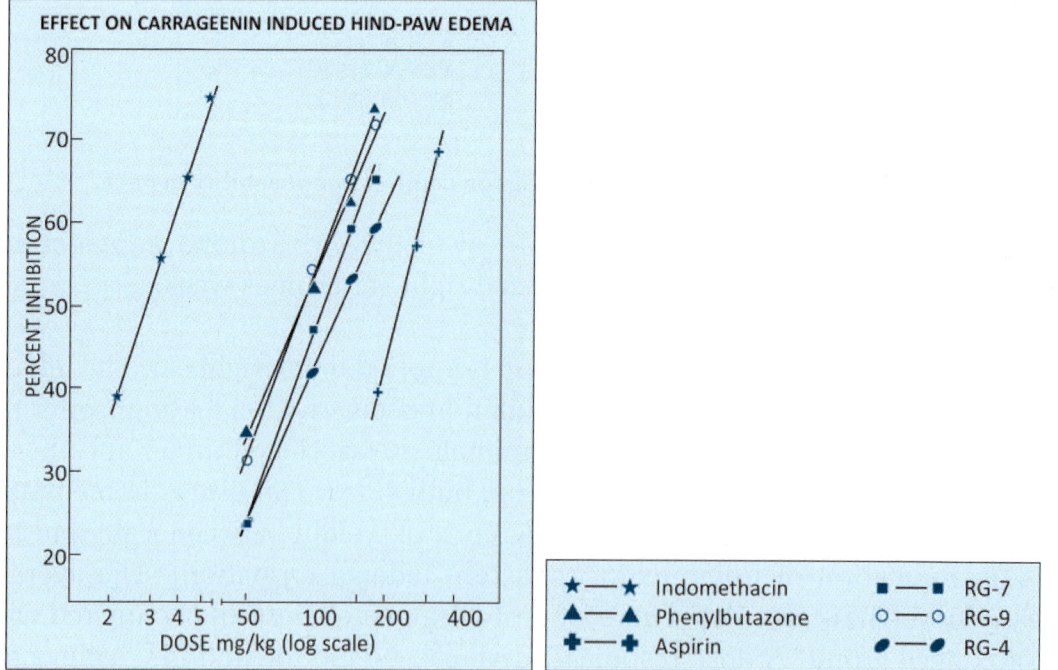

Fig. 7.5: Effect of anti-inflammatory drugs on carrageenan-induced hind paw edema in rats.

inhibition of edema formation by comparing with that of vehicle treated control animals. The average values between treated and control group is calculated for each time interval and analyzed statistically. The percent inhibition of edema formation is calculated using formula:

% inhibition = Vc – Vt/Vt × 100, where Vc is the mean paw edema volume in control group and Vt is the mean paw edema volume in test group. Dose response curve is plotted (doses against percent inhibition of edema formation).

The various phlogistic agents mentioned earlier can also be used for evaluating anti-inflammatory activity.

Cotton-pellet induced granuloma (sub-chronic inflammation)

Albino rats of Wistar strain weighing 120-150 g are used. Rats are randomely divided (6-8 rats/group) into various groups as per the experimental design. Rats are anaesthetized with ether anaesthesia and 4 sterilized Cotton-pellet (10 mg) are implanted on either side (2 on each side) of ventral region by making small subcutaneous incision. The incisions are sutured by sterile catgut. Animals are treated on the same day with test drug and reference drug daily orally for 8 days. Control rats are treated with vehicle for similar number of days. On the 9th day, 24

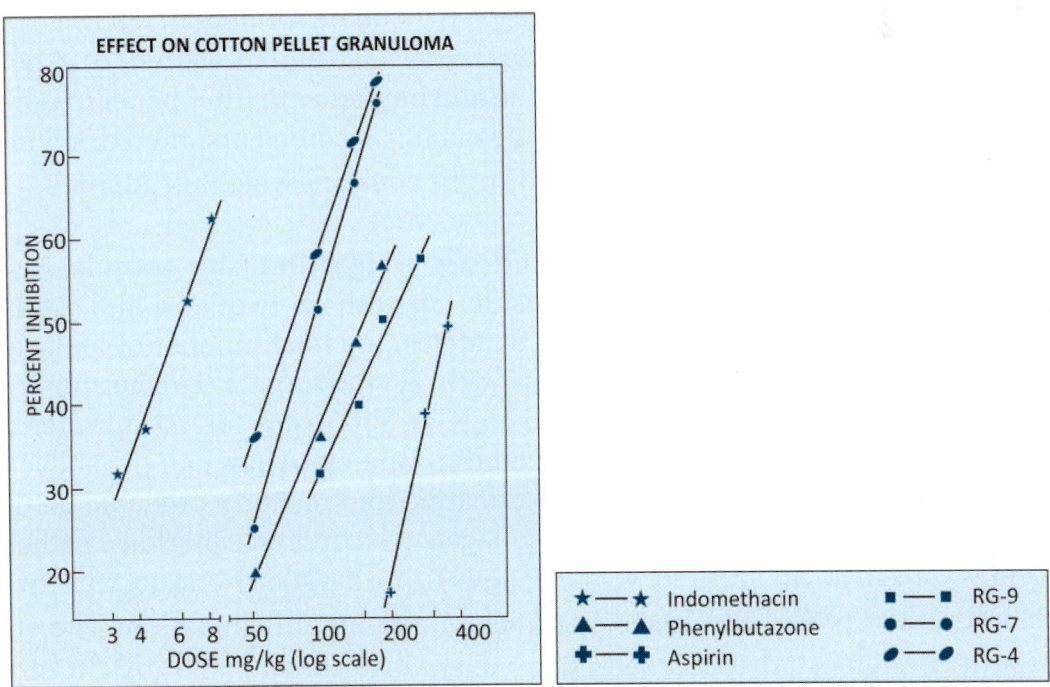

Fig.7.6: Effect of anti-inflammatory drugs on Cotton Pellet Granuloma.

hour after the last dose, the rats are anaesthetized with ether anaesthesia and sacrificed. Cotton-pellets are carefully removed and freed from extraneous tissues. Each pellet is subsequently dried at $55 \pm 5°C$ in an oven for 6 hours or until constant weight is attained. The net dry weight (i.e. wet weight-dry weight of the cotton pellet) that largely represents granular tissue formation. Prior to sacrifice the blood is withdrawn by cardiac puncture for the determination of various biochemical parameters. Even some vital tissues/organs are separated for critical biochemical studies. A dose response curve can be plotted dose versus percentage inhibition of dry weight of granuloma. ED_{50} dose can also be calculated for the determination of efficacy of the drug in cotton pellet granuloma.

Granuloma Pouch method (subchronic inflammation)

Granuloma pouch can be prepared in rats by injecting different irritants viz croton oil, turpentine, carrageenan and alpha-tocopherol into the pouch (which is prepared by injecting subcutaneously 25 ml of air on the dorsal side shaved with the help of electric clipper) of the rat. Granuloma pouch method (air pouch model) helps to determine the potency of anti-inflammatory activity by using biological parameters such as volume of exudation and granuloma tissue formation.

The test compound is injected directly into the pouch along with the irritant (separately). Due to local irritant effect leads to exudate formation. On the 8th day the pouch is opened carefully and exudates is collected and measured. Also pouch is removed and washed with normal saline and blotted with filter paper to remove excess of normal saline. Wet weight of the pouch is recorded and then dried in the oven at $55 \pm 5°C$ in an oven for 6 hours or until constant weight is attained.

The difference between wet weight and dry weight indicate granular tissue formation. Drug effect is evaluated considering both on exudates and granular tissue formation parameters. In this the exudates, the total number of leukocytes migrated can be quantified by staining with Erythrosine B. Furthermore, the exudates is centrifuged in a cold centrifuge at 3000 rpm for 10 minutes and biochemical parameters such as prostaglandins and cytokines can be assayed in order to understand the etiology of inflammation and to study probable mode of action of drugs. In the granular tissue, collagen, mucopolysaccharides, catheptic enzymes can also be studied with a view to understand connective tissue metabolism and role of lysosomal enzymes in chronic inflammation. The effect of test drug/reference drug on such parameters may throw some insight on the mechanism of drug.

Pleurisy animal model

Pleurisy can be induced in animals by using several irritants (such as histamine, bradykinin, prostaglandin, mast cell degranulator, dextran, enzymes, antigens, microbes, turpentine and carrageenan).

Carrageenan induced pleurisy is generally considered to be an excellent model in which fluid extravasation, leukocyte migration and many biochemical parameters involved in the inflammatory response can easily be measured in the exudates.

Either mouse or rats can be used in this test, and pleurisy can be induced by single injection of 0.1 ml of carrageenan (1% w/v) into pleural cavity. Animals are sacrificed 8 hours after under anesthetic ether, thorax is opened and the pleurisy cavity is washed with 1 ml of sterile phosphate buffer saline (PBS) containing heparin (20 IU per ml) samples of pleural lavage is collected for the assay of, myeloperoxidase, adenosine-deaminase activities and nitric oxide levels as well as the determination of total and differential leukocyte counts in the exudates. Such biochemical studies helps to understand under lying mechanism(s) of inflammation.

The cytospin preparations of pleural wash were stained with May-Grunwald Giemsa for the differential leukocyte counts which are generally carried out under oil immersion objective. The serum levels of C-reactive protein can also be analyzed. The values of each experimental group are averaged and compared with that of the control group. ED_{50} values are also calculated using different doses of test compound and reference drug.

Urate crystal induced inflammation (Gouty arthritis):

Urate crystals are employed to study the acute phase of the inflammatory reactions. In this method, inflammation is induced in the right rear foot pad of rats by injecting 0.1 ml of 2% sodium urate crystals in saline, the left foot of the animal serving as control. This method is more suitable for the evaluation of anti-gout agents. The edema is measured using plethysmometer by volume displacement method. The percent inhibition of edema is calculated by comparing with that of control groups using the formula mentioned earlier. A dose response curve is plotted and ED_{50} is calculated. The potency of the test compound is determined by comparing with the groups treated with standard anti-inflammatory/anti-gout drugs.

Some researchers injected sodium urate and ellagic acid into the synovial space of the stifle joint of the dog and measured synovial fluid, and pressure exerted by the appropriate foot for the development of pain. This method is more reliable and widely acceptible for comparing the relative potencies of anti-inflammatory drugs as well as anti-gout agents.

Urate induced inflammation in Pigeon:

The method is based on the measurement of delay onset of standing on one leg by pigeon after an intra-tarsal injection of talc suspension or Urate crystal. Method seems to be reliable to study the anti-inflammatory/anti-gout drug activity.

Chick embryo technique:

This method involves placing a filter paper disc on chorio-allantoic membrane of the eight day old chick embryo, incubating at 37°C for 4 days and measuring the inflammatory reaction on the adjacent membrane. This method is used for studying localized inflammatory reaction. Some drug/extract inhibit membrane irritation on the chick chorio-allantoic membrane and thus, inhibit localized inflammation. This model is also used to quantify angiogenesis induced by inflammatory effector molecules being specialized, highly vascularized tissue of the avian embryo.

Experimental arthritis model (Chronic inflammation):

Arthritis is an autoimmune disorder characterized by pain, swelling and stiffness and immobility of various joints. It is an inflammation of synovial joint due to immune mediated responses.

Table 7.1: Models of Experimentally-induced arthritis in rodents

Model	Rat/Mouse	Examples of arthritogens
Adjuvant induced arthritis (AA)	Rat	Heat-killed *M. tuberculosis* H37Ra or smegmatis
Antigen induced arthritis (AA)	Mouse/Rat	Methylated bovine serum (BSA)
Avridine induced arthritis	Rat	Avridine (CP20961)
Collagen induced arthritis	Mouse/Rat	Type II collagen

Model	Rat/Mouse	Examples of arthritogens
Immune-complex mediated arthritis (ICA)	Mouse	Antigen and the corresponding antibody
GPI induced arthritis	Mouse	Glucose-6-phosphate isomerase
Pristane induced arthritis	Mouse /Rats	Pristane
Proteoglycan induced arthritis	Mouse	Cartilage proteoglycan (aggregan)
Streptococcal cell-wall induced arthritis	Rat	Group ABC streptococci

Table 7.2: Models of Spontaneously developing arthritis

Mouse model	Arthritogenic effector mechanism
IL-1Ra knockout	Genetic deficiency of IL-1 receptor antagonist (IL-1Ra)
IL-6R knockin	Tyrosine to phenylalanine point mutation in GP130 subunit of IL-6 receptor causes enhanced IL-6 signaling
Inducible Jun knockout	Detection of june B and C-jun protein in keratinocytes using cre-lox system leads to increase in chemokine production
K/BxN	Cross-reactive autoantibodies against glucose-6 phosphate isomerase (GPI)
SKG	A defective thymic selection of T cells due to a mutation in SH2 domain of ZAP70
TNF alpha transgenic	Increased TNF-alpha production

Formalin-induced arthritis:

Formalin (2.5%) 0.1 ml/paw injected subcutaneously into the subplantar region of the hind paws of rats on 1st and 3rd day. The rats were administered with the test compound and reference drug from the first day onwards daily for 10 days. The hind paw volumes of rats are measured using digital plethysmometer by volume displacement method, 2 hours after the drug treatment. On 1st, 5th, 8th and 10th day, the percent inhibition of the hind paw edema formations is calculated using the formula mentioned below:

% inhibition = $(1 - Vt/Vc) \times 100$

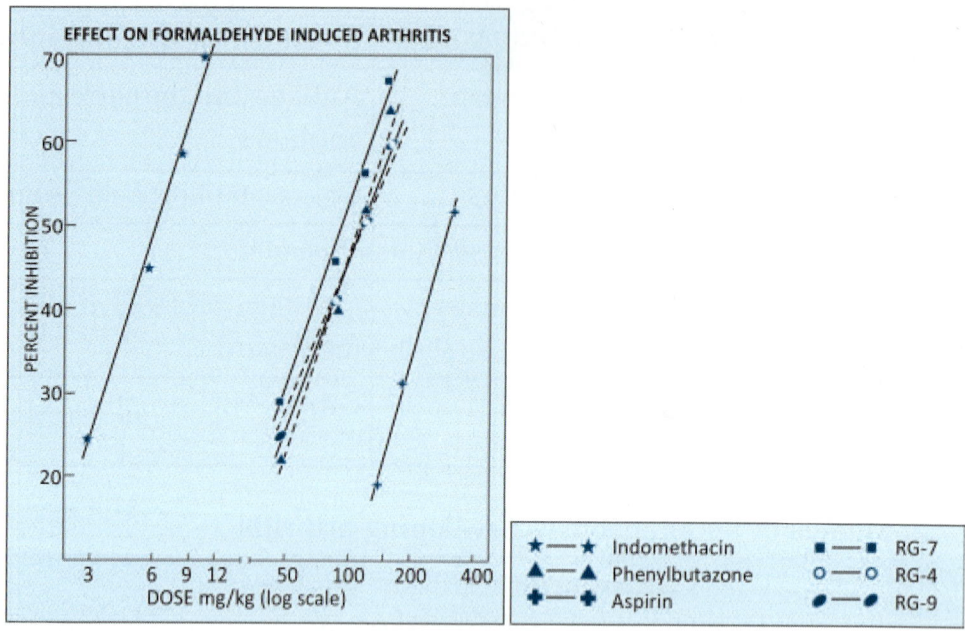

Fig. 7.7: Effect of anti-inflammatory drugs on formaldehyde induced arthritis in rats.

Vc is the mean paw edema in control group and Vt is the mean paw edema volume in test group.

Some researchers also measure the diameter of the ankle joints. The decrease in diameter is considered to be inhibition of joint inflammation. The other pharmacological parameters for arthritic index considered are hind paw edema, mobility of ankle joints, diameter of ankle joints and nociceptive response threshold. On the 10th day X-rays of the ankle joints and hind legs of the rats are taken under mild anaesthesia for the assessment of possible bone, cartilage and other structural degeneration.

Complete Freund adjuvant-induced arthritis:

Treatment schedule of Freund's adjuvant arthritis (During Arthritis development)

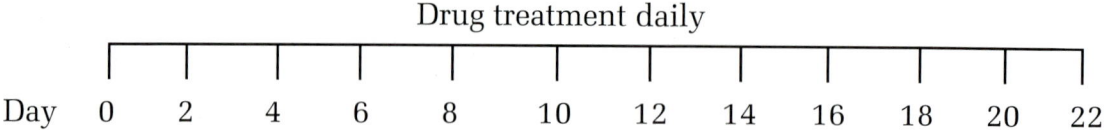

Freund's adjuvant injection, recording of Paw edema and parameters for scoring system

Treatment schedule of Freund's adjuvant arthritis (Established Arthritis)

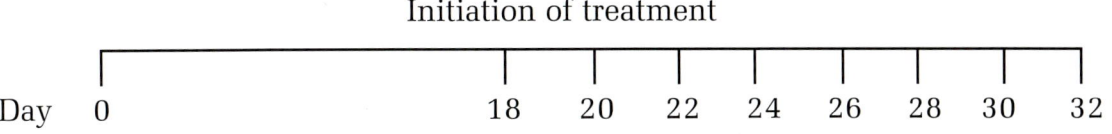

Initiation of treatment

| Day | 0 | | 18 | 20 | 22 | 24 | 26 | 28 | 30 | 32 |

Freund's adjuvant injection, recording of Paw edema and other parameters for scoring system.

Rats are injected 0.1 ml/paw of 2 mg/ml of complete Freund's adjuvant (sigma-aldrich chemicals, USA) subcutaneously into the plantar region of the right hind paw on the 1st and 7th day. Hind paw volumes of rats were measured using digital plethysmometer on 3rd, 5th, 8th, 12th, 16th and 21st day. The percent inhibition of paw edema of each group of (normal and treated with different drugs) rats is calculated using the formula as described earlier.

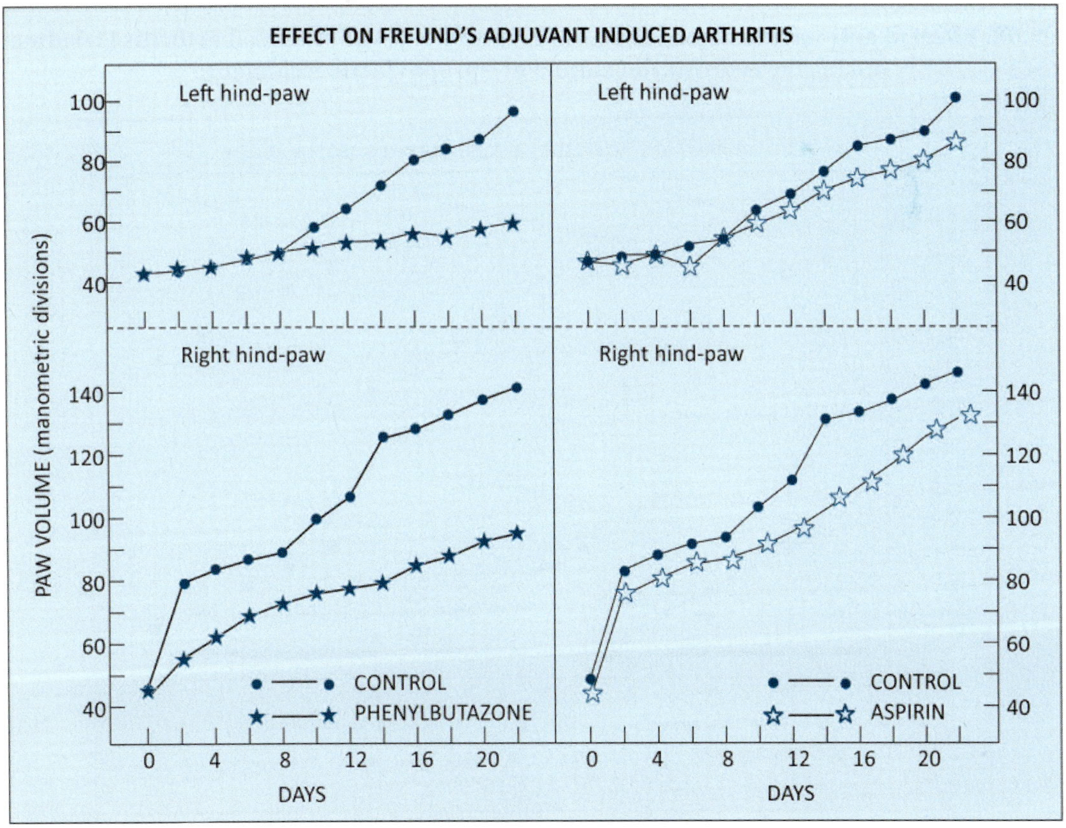

Fig 7.8A: Effect of anti-inflammatory drugs on Freund's adjuvant induced arthritis (Treatment during the arthritic development – prophylactic treatment).

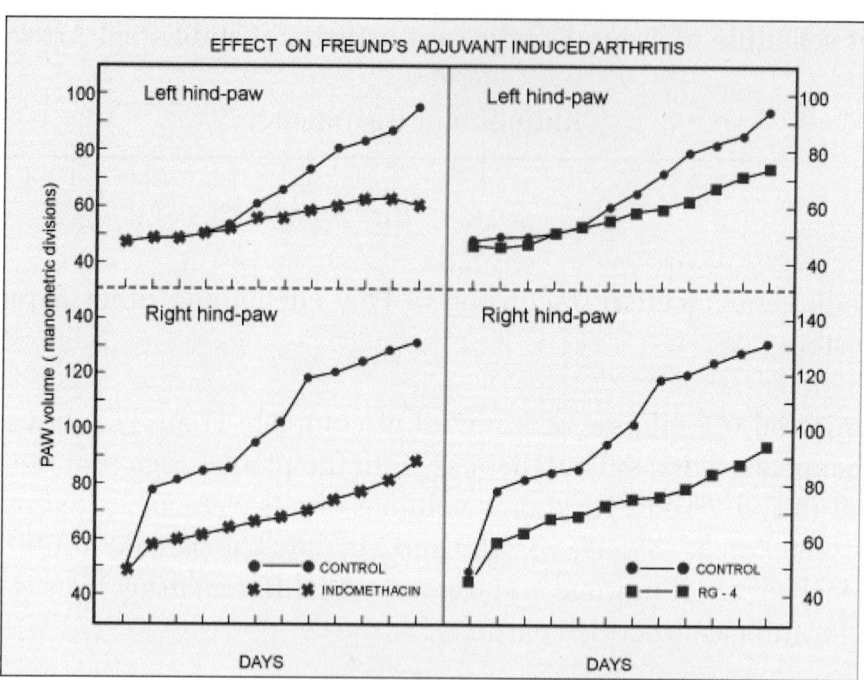

Fig. 7.8B: Effect of anti-inflammatory drugs on Freund's adjuvant induced arthritis (Treatment during the arthritic development – prophylactic treatment).

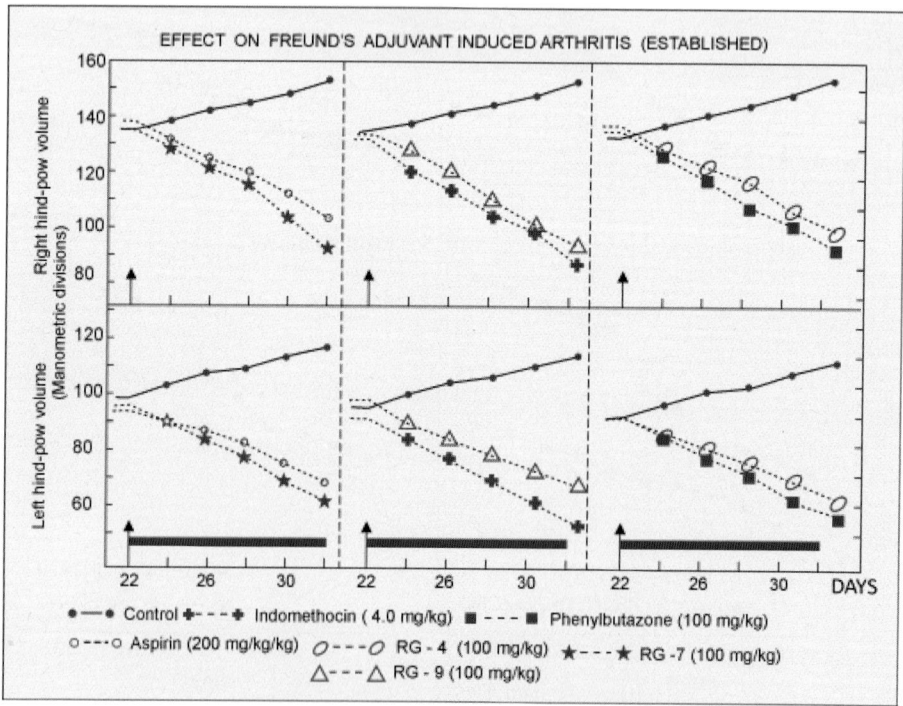

Fig. 7.9: Effect of anti-inflammatory drugs Freund's adjuvant induced arthritis (Established-therapeutic treatment).

Hind paw volumes of rats were measured using digital plethysmometer on 18th, 20th, 22nd, 24th, 26th, 28th, 30th and 32nd day.

Arthritic index is determined using various parameters, with following scoring system.

Arthritic index of rats were determined on day 3rd, day 7th, day 10th and 21st day. The evaluation of drug effect is normally carried out during arthritis development (prophylaxis treatment) and also on the established arthritis (therapeutic treatment) in this case treatment starts on the 18th day onwards for 15 days.

Arthritic index scoring system:
Primary lesion (injected paw)	1
Secondary lesion (uninjected paw)	2
1. Pinna nodules	3
2. Tail nodules	4

Motility of joints is assessed by moving ankle joints for 4 times, squeak response for pain in each ankle joint movement is counted.
Four squeak, (1) two squeaks (2), for one squeak (3) and no squeak (4)

Grip strength of hind limbs are measured by keeping the rats upright down on an inclined plane (wire mesh) and scored on the basis of latency time for sliding down, immediately (0), sliding down within 1 minute (1), sliding down within 2 minutes (2) or more than 3 minutes (3) or maintaining by holding wire mesh more than 3 minutes (4). Percent inhibition of hind paws edema and reduction of ankle diameter is also considered for arthritic index.

Proteoglycan induced arthritis

Proteoglycan aggrecan (PG), a major macromolecular component of cartilage is highly immunogenic, it induces arthritis in genetically susceptible BALB/c mice. PG core protein-specific synthetic peptide is used for priming as well as hyper immunizing BALB/c mice.

High buoyant density cartilage proteoglycans (PG) are prepared from fetal and adult human, canine or bovine articular cartilage as well as 1 week old mouse epiphysal cartilage. 100 μg of deglycosylated proteinglycan protein is injected intraperitoneally on day 0, 21st and 42nd. The first injection is with complete Freund's adjuvant, whereas second and third booster contained antigen in-complete Freund's adjuvant. Typically PG-immunized susceptible BALB/c mice develop arthritis in 10-14 days after the last booster dose. Animals are treated with the test drug or vehicle from 20-40 days. Sera from mice with progressive polyarthritis is tested for antibodies to arthritogenic proteoglycan during week 12-18 of immunization.

Besides these models there are number of experimental models of rheumatoid arthritis are used to study pathogenesis and to understand the fundamental mechanisms of underpinning rheumatoid arthritis. The substances used for induction of arthritis model include collagen induced arthritis and the methylated BSA model and genetically manipulated or spontaneous arthritis such as TNF alpha-transgenic mouse, K/BxN mouse and SKG mouse. Some of these models are described **(Table 7.1 and 7.2)**. Some of these models have proven invaluable to unravel the pathophysiological pathways of inflammatory arthritis and for investigational testing of therapeutic agents.

Biochemical Properties of Anti-inflammatory drugs

1) The role of polypeptides and amines derived by decarboxylation of alpha-amino acids in inflammatory reactions has been documented, and non-steroidal drugs inhibit decarboxylase. For exemple, histidine decarboxylase, glutamine dehydrogenase, transaminases and many more enzymes are also associated with decarboxylation and peptide breakdown process.

2) The connective tissue constituent's viz. mucopolysaccharides, d-glucose amine, d-galactosamine are altered during inflammation. Many anti-inflammatory drugs of both steroidal and non-steroidal are reported to inhibit 2enzyme system which carry out amination in granular tissue, synovial tissue, bovine heart valves and cartilage.

   Many anti-inflammatory drugs inhibit ATP formation in tissues and also suppress glucose utilization by extrahepatic and other tissues causing inhibition of inflammation/edema formation.

3) Mucopolysaccharides profoundly influence the structure, rigidity and state of hydration of body's supporting tissues and joint fluid as well. Many of the anti-inflammatory drugs of steroidal and non-steroidal origin known to inhibit mucopolysaccharide biosynthesis in connective tissues, collagen formation in granulation tissue, skin and cartilage. Hydroxyproline may be an excellent parameter to study the collagen metabolism. Most of the anti-inflammatory

drugs inhibit hydroxyproline in connective tissue. Uncoupling of oxidative phosphorylation, that selectively depress mitochondrial ATP biosynthesis leading to reduced synthesis of large intracellular molecules such as glycogen and protein together with an increased catabolism of substances already present in the cells. This is likely to interfere with selective permeability of cellular membrane across the membranes that depend on the availability of ATP. The decrease in ATP lead to diminution in the intracellular osmotic pressure accompanied by weakening of the barriers to exit and entry of fluid and electrolytes between the body cells, and their environment. Many anti-inflammatory drugs are known to induce uncouple the oxidative phosphory-lation. The uncoupling of oxidative phosphorylation may also activate ATPase in the mitochondria. Most of the anti-inflammatory drugs reported to activate selectively ATPase activity in granular tissue by repeated administration.

Anti-inflammatory drugs also inhibit dehydrogenases by competing with pyridine nucleotide coenzymes for binding site on the enzyme and may be one of the mechanism responsible for anti-inflammatory activity.

Lysosomal enzymes, acid phosphatase, lactic dehydrogenase, B-glucuronidase, cationic proteinase play important role in inflammation, paw edema and arthritis, tissue injury and breakdown of connective tissue. Most of the anti-inflammatory drugs known to stabilize the isolated lysozymes (*in-vitro*) and inhibit the release of lysosomal enzymes.

The denaturation (modification of the secondary, tertiary or quaternary structure of protein molecules, but does not involve breaking of bond). The denaturation of bovine serum albumin induced by heat, guanidine and sodium dodecyl sulphate, and measured the changes of aggregation and configuration by turbidity, viscosity and optical rotation. It was found that non-steroidal drugs inhibit the heat denaturation of bovine serum albumin, also diminish both solubility loss and viscosity rise, suggesting that drug may act at the molecular level through the changes in protein conformation. The anti-inflammatory drugs also inhibit erythrocyte lysis induced by heat and hypotonic hemolysis (*in-vitro*) which may be due to stabilization of the red cell membrane, by common properties.

The anti-inflammatory activity of non-steroidal anti-inflammatory (NSAID) drugs is mainly mediated through inhibition of biosynthesis of prostaglandins. The selectivity of COX_1 versus COX_2 is often variable and incomplete, especially for older generation of NSAIDs, but subsequently, more selective COX_2 inhibitors have been developed. Some NSAIDs inhibit both COX_1 and COX_2 but their degree of inhibition especially COX_2 is to a lesser extent. Inhibition of release of prostaglandins is the mechanism of action of anti-inflammatory corticosteroids (inhibiting phospholipase-A of the membrane phospholipids). The presence of increased reactive oxygen species (ROS) at the site of inflammation, lead to believe that oxidative stress plays a key role in the induction of rheumatoid arthritis. Anti-inflammatory drugs decrease the free radical formation including pleiotropic short lived free radical, nitric oxide (NO), superoxide dismutase (SOD) and known to damage cellular element in cartilage and extracellular matrix directly or indirectly. Such antioxidant properties are therapeutically useful in protecting tissue injury (ischemia, inflammation and hypoxia) from ROS and superoxide anions. Anti-inflammatory drugs restore the depleted antioxidant enzymes (SOD, catalase, glutathione peroxidase) and glutathione responsible for maintaining cells in reduced state, and indirectly participate in cell protection against oxidative stress. Myeloperoxidase (MPO) is the index of neutrophil infiltration. It causes lysosome destruction by dent of increase in array of ROS, which in turn upregulates hydroxyl and peroxide radicals leading to damage of tissue membranes. These events are inhibited by NSAIDs and cortisone and produce anti-inflammatory effect. Leukocytes, including neutrophils, macrophages and fibroblasts are the primary source of cytokines. The synovial macrophages and fibroblasts produce plethora of proinflammatory cytokines (interleukins, TNF-alpha and chemokines). Among these interleukins, IL-1b, IL-6 and TNF-alpha are found to be most active mediators and participates in the pathogenesis and progression of arthritis. The NSAIDs, steroid hormones and disease modifying anti-rheumatic drugs (Methotrexate, Cyclosporine are also known to produce significant therapeutic effect in arthritis models.

Significant increase of polyamines (putrescine, spermidine and spermine) in the inflamed tissue in both acute and chronic inflammation has been documented. Treatment with dexamethasone and polyamines themselves shown to elicit significant anti-inflammatory activity both in acute and chronic inflammation, and their effects are attributed due to their antioxidant and/or lysosomal membrane stabilization properties.

Analgesic drug screening methods in animals

The problem of ascertaining whether a chemical entity has the ability to relieve pain or not in animals has been a perplexing one for the experimental pharmacologist. A large number of experimental methods and designs that have been developed during past 4-5 decades, are reflections of the difficulties inherent in the problem. A potentially noxious stimulus in the animal will evoke reflex response when pain threshold has been reached and most of these reflexes have been used as indicators of the character of stimulus (reaction time). Many of the reflexes are of escape nature. e.g. tail flick, skin twitches, limb flexion, squeak, licking paws. Such reflexes have formed the basis for determining the "pain threshold" in animals, and analgesic drugs are screened by testing their ability to raise such threshold. Bias of the observer during experiment can be overcome by a proper selection of an experimental design.

Tail clip method

In this method mice weighing between 20-25 g body weights are used. A bull dog clip is applied to the base of the tail of the mouse and reaction is recorded in seconds from the time the clip is applied until the animal tried to remove it. Mice not responding within 5 seconds to this mechanical stimulus are discarded. Prolongation of reaction time beyond 10 seconds is considered to indicate analgesic action.

Hot plate method

A hot plate is maintained 55±0.5°C. The mouse is placed on the hot plate and the time was recorded in seconds until the mouse starts either licking the front paws or jumped out of plastic cylinder placed on the hot plate. Normal mice react to thermal stimulus within 5 seconds. When the reaction time is increased by 8 seconds or more, it is considered that the test drug has analgesic action.

Electric shock method

Electric shock (voltage 25.0, pulse width 20 seconds, frequency 1/sec) is applied through a square wave stimulator to the tail of the mouse and number of shocks which caused the animal to squeak are counted. If a medicated mouse required more than 3 shocks or above the pre-drug number, it is considered that the test compound possess analgesic activity.

All drugs are given orally or intraperitoneally. The intervals between the injection of pre drug treatment and the induction to painful stimulus (mechanical, thermal or electrical) are performed as per the experimental protocol/design of the experiment. Generally the drugs must produce analgesic action within the shortest possible period, may be within 15 minutes and the effect should persist for longer time period. Hence analgesic tests are carried out 15, 30, 60 and 120 min after the drug treatment. Control group mice are treated with normal saline or vehicle used for the preparation of the test drug. Reference drugs such as (aspirin, paracetamol) non-narcotics-peripherally acting drugs or narcotic drugs (like morphine, meperidine or codeine are used) which are acting on the central nervous system are used as reference standard. A dose response effect can be studied, and ED_{50} of drug can also be determined by the method of Litchfield and Wilcoxon (1949).

Writing method

Mice and rats are used for this experiment. Test drugs are administered orally, and 30 minutes later 0.1 ml/10g of 0.3% v/v acetic acid solution is injected intraperitoneally. The writhing episodes such as "stretching of hind limbs" and "bending of abdomen" are counted during 30 minutes following the acetic acid injection and are selected. Forty eight hours later, the selected mice are randomly divided into different groups as per test drug treatment schedule (doses) and reference drug. Each group consists of 6-8 mice/group. Non-narcotic analgesics block this reaction but so do local anesthetics, antihistamines and large number of compounds belong to different category. The percentage of analgesic activity of test drug is assessed by decrease in writhing episodes as compared to control group. Dose response effect curve (percentage protection versus doses) is plotted or ED_{50} for each drug can be calculated by the method of Litchfield and Wilcoxon (1949) to evaluate potency of test compounds.

$$\text{The percentage protection} = \frac{\text{Number of writhing episodes in treated animals}}{\text{Number of writhing episodes in control group}} \times 100$$

Tail flick method

Rats or mice are used for this experiment. The tail flick method is performed on (dolorimeter) analgesiometer. General principle of applying sharply localized heat to induce a response from animals has been more widely adopted in various dolorimeter. The temperature of the analgesiometer is maintained at 55±0.5°C. The reaction time in seconds is used as a unit for measurement of pain and increase in reaction time is the indication of analgesia. The time of placing the tail of the rat/mouse on the radiant heat source (the nichrome wire which is heated and temperature 55°C is maintained by water circulation) and sharp withdrawal of the tail is recorded as "reaction time". Cut off time of 10 seconds is considered as maximum latency so as to avoid the thermal injury while recording the reaction

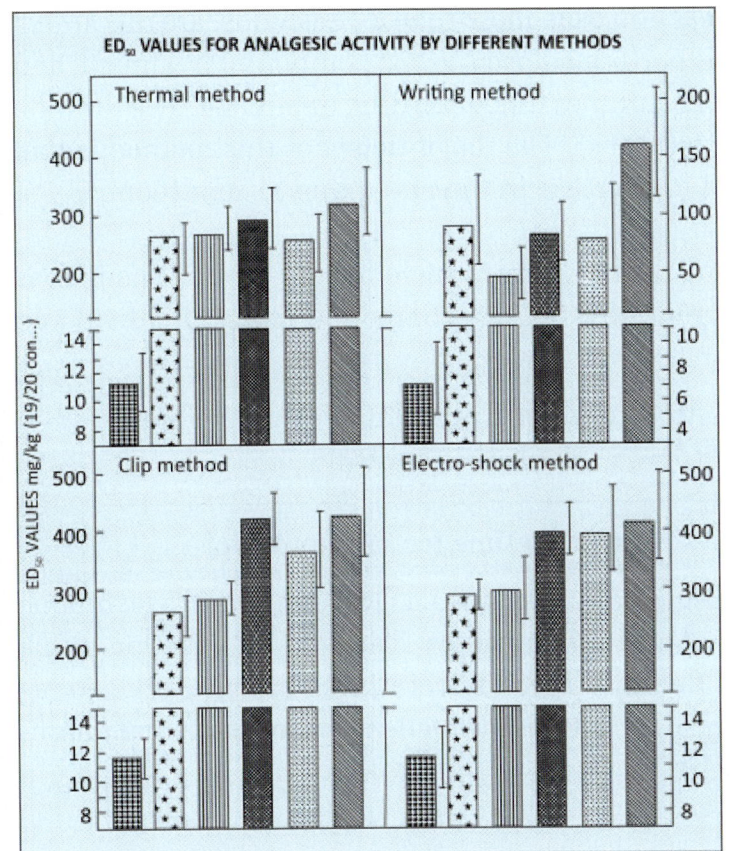

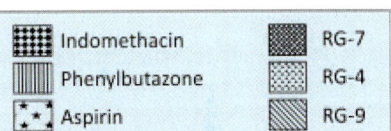

Fig. 7.10: ED$_{50}$ values for analgesic activity by different methods.

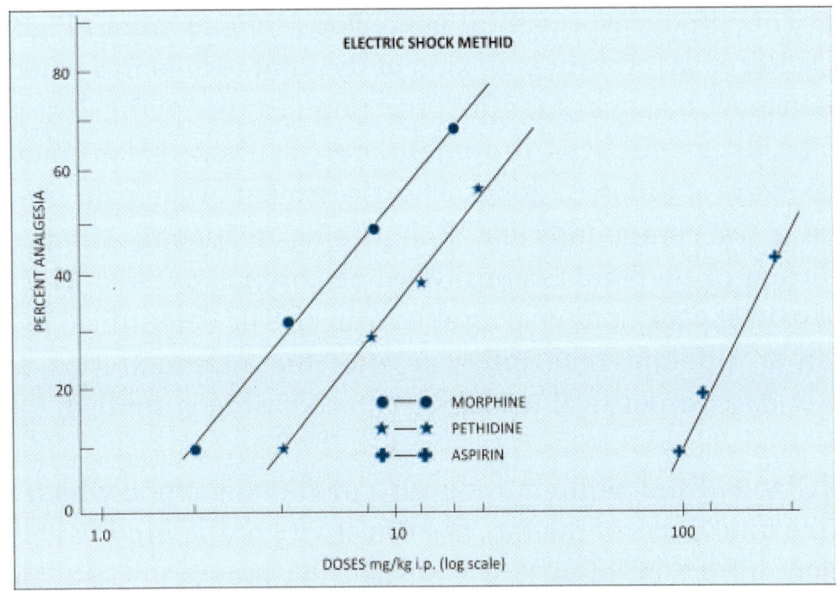

Fig. 7.11: Electric shock method.

time. Rats/mice show a mean reaction time more than 5-6 seconds, are discarded. In all groups, tail flick method is performed prior to test compound treatment, and thereafter at 15, 30, 60, 90 and 120 minutes following drug treatment. The reaction time at each time interval is determined. The major defect of this method is that repeated use of the animal lead to decrease in threshold due to conditioning.

Compare results of treated group with control vehicle treated group. The ED_{50} is calculated by taking three different doses of test compound using Litchfield and Wilcoxin's method.

$$\text{Analgesia in percentage} = \frac{\text{Reaction time for treatment - reaction time for saline control}}{\text{Reaction time for saline control}} \times 100$$

Randall and Selito (1967) and Segmaund, Cadmus Lu (1957) reported a technique which demonstrates the effect of anti-inflammatory drugs on the reaction to the inflammatory pain induced by the injection of silver nitrate into the ankle joints of rats because pain and inflammatory actions normally represent different phases of a single phenomenon.

Silver Nitrate method

This test is performed in rats. Rats are injected 0.1 ml of silver nitrate (1%) into ankle joints. This produces a painful edematous inflammation. Eighteen hours after the injection of silver nitrate, flexion of the joint results in a painful reaction that is accompanied by squeak (animal reaction towards pain). Test compounds and reference drugs such as Indomethacin, aspirin, phenylbutazone are administered orally at different doses. The assessment of the pain is made before the treatment of test compounds and 5 hours after treatment. Absence of squeak on abrupt flexion of the joint is considered as absence of pain. The percentage inhibition of pain at peak hour of drug effect can also be determined by measuring pain reaction at different time intervals after the administration of drug/test compounds. A dose response at peak hour effect of drug is studied.

Susequently, Randall and Selito introduced a modified method which applies the pressure to the hind paws of the rat. The sensitivity of the hind paw is increased by the injection of 0.1 ml of 20% w/v suspension brewer's yeast. Threshold in inflamed paw is increased not only by narcotic drugs but also by sodium salicylate and phenylbutazone. This method though sensitive enough as there is a lack of strict correlation between the amount of edema and the degree of hyperesthesia in the paw edema. Aspirin in regular dose having no significant effect on paw edema volume, but there is a marked increase in the reaction threshold for squeak response.

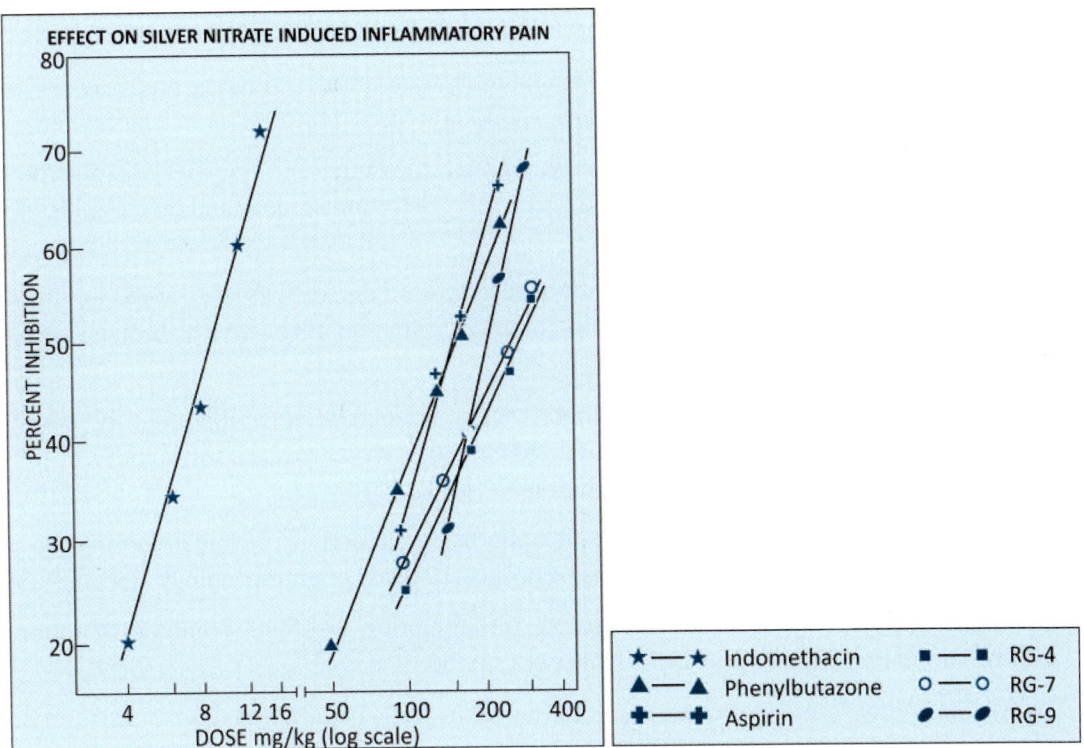

Fig. 7.12: Effect of Silver Nitrate induced inflammatory pain.

References:

1. Atul T. Thite, Rajesh R Patil and Suresh Ramnath Naik (2014). Anti-arthritic activity profile of methanolic extract of Ficusbengalensis: Comparison with some clinically effective drugs. Biomed & Aging Pathol 4, 207-217.

2. Bradford et al (2017): Animal models of rheumatoid pain experimental system and insights. Arthritis Research & Therapy 19:146

3. Chakradhar, V., and Suresh Ramnath Naik. "Polyamines in inflammation and their modulation by conventional anti-inflammatory drugs." (2007).

4. Delaunay, A., and S. Bazin. "Metabolic changes in connective tissue during an inflammatory process." International Symposium on Non-steroidal Anti-inflammatory Drugs, (1969) Edited by GARATTINI, S., MILAN, MNG AND DUKES, O.

5. DELAUNAY, ALBERT, and SUZANNE BAZIN. "Modification of chemical components in inflamed connective tissue." Inflammation biochemistry and drug interaction. Excerpta Medica Foundation, Amsterdam (1969): 94.

6. Kalyanpur, S.G., S.R. Naik, and U.K. Sheth 1968. "Study of biochemical effects of anti-inflammatory drugs in carrageenan induced oedema and cotton pellet granuloma." Biochemical pharmacology 17., 797.

7. Kamal, D Moudgid, Peter, Kim and Emnest Brahn MD (2011): Curr. Rheumatol Re p 13:

8. Naik, S.R., and U.K. Sheth (1976) "Inflammatory process and screening methods for anti-inflammatory agents-a review." Journal of Postgraduate Medicine 22:5.

9. Naik, S.R., and S.M. Wala (2014) "Arthritis, a complex connective and synovial joint destructive autoimmune disease: animal models of arthritis with varied etiopathology and their significance." Journal of postgraduate medicine 60, 309.

10. Naik, S.R., and U.K. Sheth (1978) "Studies on two new derivatives of N-aralkyl-o-ethoxy-benzamides: Part II—biochemical studies on their anti-inflammatory activity." Indian journal of experimental biology 16:1175.

11. Naik, S.R., S.G. Kalyanpur, and U.K. Sheth (1972). "Effects of anti-inflammatory drugs on glutathione levels and liver succinic dehydrogenase activity in carrageenin edema and cotton pellet granuloma in rats." Biochemical pharmacology 22:511.

12. Naik, S.R (1984). "Increased cyclic AMP-phosphodiesterase activity during inflammation and its inhibition by anti-inflammatory drugs." European journal of pharmacology 104: 253-259.

13. Vane, J. O. H. N., and Regina Botting. (1987) "Inflammation and the mechanism of action of anti-inflammatory drugs." The FASEB journal 1: 89-96.

14. Winter, C., E. Risley, and O. Nuss (1962). "Carrageenin-induced inflammation in the hind limb of the rat." FEDERATION PROCEEDINGS, 1962.

15. Weissman G. (1966): Lysosomes and joint diseases. Arthr and Rheum 9, 834-840.

16. Grewal, RS (1952): A method for testing analgesia in mice. Brit J Pharmard 1,433-437.

17. Whitehouse, M.W., and J.M. Haslam (1962) "Ability of some antirheumatic drugs to uncouple oxidative phosphorylation." Nature 196.: 1323-1324.

18. Whitehouse, M.W., and H. Boström (1962). "The effect of some anti-inflammatory (anti-rheumatic) drugs on the metabolism of connective tissues." Biochemical pharmacology 11.: 1175-1201.

19. Witkin, L.B., et al. (1961) "Pharmacology of 2-amino-indane hydrochloride (Su-8629): a potent non-narcotic analgesic." Journal of Pharmacology and Experimental Therapeutics 133.3 (1961): 400-408.

20. WOOLFE, GAND, and A.D. MacDonald. (1944) "The evaluation of the analgesic action of pethidine hydrochloride (Demerol)." Journal of Pharmacology and Experimental Therapeutics 80.: 300-307.

8 ANTI-ALLERGIC AND ANTI-ASTHMATIC DRUGS SCREENING METHODS

Allergy can be broadly defined as a damaging response(s) or reaction(s) by the body to a particular substance, especially a particular food, pollen, fur, insects bite, ticks or moulds, to which it has become hyper-sensitive that lead to reactions that manifest in symptoms like inflammation (redness and swelling), allergic rhinitis, conjunctivitis (eye), eczema, hives (urticaria), asthma (lungs). This hyper-sensitivity reaction has been largely mediated by histamine initially. Following antigen- antibody reaction on their surface (IgE type of antigenic antibodies) mast cells are released in immediate type hypersensitivity reactions. Such situations make a person sick or develop breathing problems, diarrhea, fall in blood pressure etc. In these reactions first sensitization occurs upon initial encounter with antigen, and effectors phase involves immunogenic memory and causes tissue damage either subsequent interaction with specific antigen. Three types of hypersensitivity reactions are mediated by antibodies:

Type I Hypersensitivity reaction - This is an immediate hypersensitivity mediated by IgE and symptoms are manifested within few minutes after the interaction with antigen. Generally such reactions occur mainly due to cross-linkage of membrane- bound IgE on blood basophils or tissue mast cells by antigen, releasing histamine, leukotriene and eosinophil chemotactic factor.

Type II Hypersensitivity reaction - This type of reactions occurs due to the formation of complexes between antigen with antibodies (IgM or IgG). Similar type of reactions occurs during blood transfusion (if blood is not corrected cross matching) and penicillin induced allergy. Mediation of hypersensitivity reactions has been initially dissociated with histamine, released from mast cells following antigen- antibody reaction on their surface, by IgE type antibodies in the immediate type of hypersensitivity reaction (type 1). Histamine is known to cause urticaria, angioedema bronchoconstriction and anaphylactic reaction. The other likely mediators are: leukotriene (LTD-4), platelet activating factor etc.

117

Type III Hypersensitivity reaction - Type III hypersensitivity reactions has been largely attributed to the deposition of immune complexes that lead to activation of components (C5a, C3a and C4a) that can cause serious anaphylatoxic and chemotactic activities which finally manifest in increased vascular permeability and recruitment of neutrophils. The major chemical symptoms are skin rashes, glomerulonephritis and arthritis.

Type IV Hypersensitivity reaction (Delayed type hypersensitivity) - This is cell mediated hypersensitivity reaction occurs 2-4 days after the exposure of sensitizing antigen. This causes local edema, tissue damage due to non-specific, non-inflammatory macrophages by specific Th1 cells. Delayed type hypersensitivity are extremely useful in eliminating interactions caused by intracellular pathogens, (mycobacterium tuberculosis and leishmania strains).

A. Anti-allergy Drug Screening Methods (*In-vivo*):

1. **Milk-induced Eosinophilia and Leukocytosis in Mice**

    It is documented that a significant increase in leukocytes and eosinophils count in rodents 24 hours after parenteral administration of milk. The eosinophils are the most characteristic inflammatory cells in bronchial biopsies taken from asthamatic patients and may be seen in submucosal and epithelial layers. The leucocytes recruited during asthmatic inflammation release the mediators like cytokines, histamine and major basic proteins that promote and sustain ongoing inflammation. Eosinophilia is defined as abnormal increase in eosinophils (more than 4% of total leukocyte count). In asthmatic patients there is a marked increase in eosinophilia counts. The involvement of eosinphil in bronchial mucosa, in which allergic inflammation occurs, is critical factor to the late asthmatic reaction and mucus hypersecretion. When these cells are recruited, they degranulate mast cells leading to histamine release that cause airway inflammation.

    Experimental Procedure: Select Swiss albino mice weighing between 25-30 gm and divide them randomly into various groups. Treat the control group of mice with vehicle [CMC (10 ml/kg, p.o.) or normal saline (10 ml/kg, p.o)]. Administer test drug (at an effective dose by i.p. / p.o.) and reference drug [Dexamethasone (0.27 mg/kg, i.p.)] to other group of mice. Maintain one group of mice without any treatment. Administer boiled and cooled cow's milk (4 ml/kg, s.c.) one hour later to all groups of mice. Withdraw the blood samples from each mouse from retro-orbital plexus under light ether anesthesia, 24 h after the milk administration. Count total leukocytes and eosinophils in blood by adding few drops of diluted blood (Using dilution fluid) on Neuber's chamber slide and under oil immersed microscope and express the results as cells per cu.mm. (Bhargava and Singh, 1981).

2. **Active anaphylaxis in rats**
    Experimental Procedure: The Wistar strain rats weighing between 200 to 250 gm are selected and divided randomly into various groups. Rats are sensitized by subcutaneously injecting 0.5 ml of horse serum along with 0.5 ml of triple antigen containing 10^4 *Bordetella pertussis.* The sensitized rats are divided into various groups (6 animals/group). Rats from normal control and positive control are administered normal saline (10 ml/kg, p.o.) daily for 10 days, whereas effective doses (based on pilot experimental findings) of test drug and reference drug are administered for similar period to the respective groups.

On the 10th day, 2 h after the last dose administration, the rats are challenged with 0.25 ml (dilute horse serum in the ratio of 1:1 in normal saline) horse serum/rat by intravenous injection. The symptoms of anaphylactic reactions, respiratory distress, increased respiratory rate, dyspnoea, cyanosis and mortality are observe and record. The severity of anaphylactic reactions especially on respiratory system is scored on a scale (0-20). The scoring system pattern is as follows: increased respiratory rate (2), dyspnoea for 10 min. (4), dyspnoea and cyanosis for 10 min (8) and respiratory collapse and death (12). Sacrifices rats 2 h after the challenge, and the intestinal mesentery is taken out for the mast cells degranulation study. Collect the mesenteries of rats along with intestinal pieces and place it in Ringer-Locke solution (NaCl 9.0, KCl 0.42, $CaCl_2$ 0.24, $NaHCO_3$ 0.15, Glucose 1.0 gm/L of distilled water at 37°C). The mesenteric pieces are challenged with 5% horse serum and allow for 10 min reactions, following which the mast cells are stained with toluidine blue and examine microscopically and count for the number of intact and granulated mast cells. Count the number of intact and disrupted mast cells in at least 10 randomly selected high power fields. Withdraw the blood from retro-orbital plexus of rats under anesthesia, and separate serum by centrifugation at 3000 rpm for 10 min. Results are expressed in terms of degree of amelioration in respiratory symptoms, and percentage protection of mast cell degranulation with standard as well as test drug. Evaluate the potency of test drug by comparing with standard drug treatment group. Use serum for the analysis of IgE and cytokine levels to understand the possible mode of action of test drug. (Mitra et al., 1999)

3. **Passive cutaneous anaphylaxis in Rats**

    Passive cutaneous anaphylaxis (PCA) is an immediate localized dermal reaction to an allergen, specifically IgE and is manifested by an enhanced permeability of vessels within the skin. To envisage and quantify the enhanced permeability, a hallmark of PCA, which is demonstrated by the intravenous injection of Evans blue, a dye that binds to and is extravated with plasma albumin. Therefore, PCA can be used as a screening model to study sensitivity to allergens and to screen the effectiveness of compound in ameliorating the reaction of anaphylaxis.

    Experimental Procedure: Administer subcutaneously (s.c) 100 mg of egg albumin (EA) + 12 mg of aluminum hydroxide to male rats on days 1, 3 and 5 for obtaining homologous rat antiserum. Withdraw the blood on the 10th day from the retro-orbital plexus under anesthesia, and separate the homologous serum by centrifugation at 3000 rpm for 10 min which contains IgE antibody. Divide the rats randomly into various groups (6 rats/group). Remove the hairs of the dorsal region of rats using electric clipper. Sensitize the rats by injecting 0.1 ml of serum intradermally on either side of the shaved dorsal area. After 48 h, administer CMC (10 ml/ kg, p.o.) to normal control group. Treat the other group of rats with test drug and reference drug. Prepare a mixture of Evans blue (0.5%) and EA (1% w/v) in normal saline and inject (0.25 ml/rat) intravenously one hour after the treatment. Thirty minutes after, mark and measure a blue color area (mm²) of the dorsal skin (antibody injected site) accurately and compare with that of control group and calculate the percentage inhibition by test and reference drug (Han et al, 2007).

    The seepage of Evans blue due to increase in capillary permeability is assayed quantitatively by removing the tissues of blue color area, homogenize in normal saline buffer, and deproteinize with 20-30% Trichloro acetic acid (TCA) solution containing 1 mM EDTA, the homogenate followed by extraction with either ethyl alcohol or methyl alcohol of the sediment. Read the absorbance of the extract at 620 nm.

4. **Delayed Type Hypersensitivity (DTH) in Mice**
    DTH is a part of the process of graft rejection, tumor immunity and immunity related many intracellular infectious microorganisms, especially those causing chronic diseases like tuberculosis. Furthermore, DTH requires the specific recognition of a given antigen for activation of lymphocytes, which subsequently proliferate and release cytokines. Such events in turn increase vascular permeability, vasodilatation, macrophage accumulation, and these events further augment increased pahgocytosis and elevation of lytic enzymes for more effective repair process. Hence, potentiating effect of DTH response suggest the stimulatory effect of test drug or standard drug on lymphocyte and other participating immune cells essential for repair process, and also augment the cell mediated immunity.

    Experimental Procedure: Randomly divide Swiss albino mice weighing 25-30 g into different groups (6 mice/group). Administer normal saline (10 ml/kg, p.o.) to normal control animals and 0.1 ml Sheep Red Blood Cells (SRBCs) (1×10^8 cells/mouse; i.p.) to positive control mice (induced control).

    Administer test and reference drug to rats daily for 5 days (i.e. from day 1 to day 5) prior to sensitization. On day 6, all mice except the normal control group mice are sensitized with the administration of 0.1 ml SRBCs (1×10^8 cell/mouse, i.p.) prepare in 0.15M phosphate buffer saline (PBS pH 7.2). After sensitization, treat all groups daily for 5 days (i.e. from day 7 to day 11) with the respective doses of test and reference drug except for the induced control group. On the 11th day, inject s.c with 1×10^8 SRBCs (50μl) into right hind footpad and 0.15M phosphate buffer saline (PBS pH 7.2) (50μl) into left hind footpad in all groups and 24 h after the last dose of test and reference drug, measure the DTH response (footpad edema) caused by hypersensitivity reaction with the help of plethysmometer in 24, 48 and 72 h after the booster injection of SRBCs, by applying the following formula.

$$\% \text{ change in foot edema} = \frac{(\text{Right footpad challenged with SRBC - Left footpad})}{\text{Left footpad}} \times 100$$

Weigh and sacrifice the mice 72 h after final footpad edema measurement under ether anesthesia, and record the weight of lyphoid organs i.e. spleen, thymus and kidney, and express as relative organ weight i.e. the ratio of organ weight to body weight.

Evaluate the drug effect on the basis of footpad edema formation. The standard drug eliciting antiallergic activity induces an enhancement of footpad edema formation in DTH mouse model. Evaluate the potency of the test drug by comparing the activity of reference drug. Drugs exhibiting anti-allergic activities produce a dose related increase in the relative weight of lymphoid organs (spleen, thymus and kidney). (Naik et al. 2009).

5. **Compound 48/80 induced mast cell degranulation in rats**

Mast cells are constituents of virtually all organs and tissues, and are important mediators of inflammatory responses, effectors cells of immediate type allergy and anaphylaxis. Mast cells derived mediators such as histamine, bradykinin and arachidonic acid are released and known potent mediators in the acute phase of immediate hypersensitivity reactions. Mast cells degranulation can be evoked by the compound 48/80 (formaldehyde polymer of p-methoxy-phenethyl-methyl-amine), and is routinely used as a direct and convenient reagent to study the mast cell stabilization aspect of drugs and to understand their probable role in producing anti-allergic activity.

The pathological mechanisms involved in Type-I allergy has been explained on the basis of the mast cells and basophils degranulation that lead to the release of mediators such as histamine, leukotrienes and prostaglandins from such cells. The compound 48/80 has been routinely used as a direct and convenient reagent to study the mechanism of allergy and anaphylaxis including mode of antiallergic activity.

Experimental Procedure: Sensitize Wistar rats (200-250 gm) by injecting of compound 48/80 (1 mg/kg of body weight by s.c.) and randomly divide into different groups (6 rats/group). Administer normal saline (10 ml/kg, p.o.) to normal control group rats while the test and reference drug (dose on the basis of experimental reports) orally or intraperitoneally to rats daily for 14 days to test and reference drug groups. Select the doses and route of test drug administration by conducting pilot experiments. On the 14th day, 2 hr after the assigned treatment, inject 10 ml of normal saline into the peritoneal cavity of rats, after gentle massage (this procedure will allow the cells to detach from tissue and transit into the phosphate buffer solution, PBS), abdomen is cut open and collect the fluid and wash the cells with Gey solution to get rid of contaminating blood till PBS is clear, and then transfer into silicones test tube containing 7-10 ml of phosphate buffer solution (pH 7.2-7.4). Purify mast cells by the method of Percoll. Wash mast cells three times by centrifugation at 4°C at low speed (1200 rpm), gently remove the cell pellet supernatant and dissolve pellets of mast cells into the solution. Incubate these cells with compound 48/80 (5 μg/ml) at 37°C for 10 min. After incubation spin and stain these cells with 0.1% toluidine blue and examine under the microscope. Count the numbers of intact and disrupted mast cells at least 10 randomly selected high power fields for each tissue. Calculate the percent protection of the reference drug by comparing its effect with that of control saline treatment group. Determine the potency of unknown/test drug by comparing its results with that of the reference drug treatment group. (Hachisuka et al. 1988).

6. **Experimentally induced Allergic rhinitis in Guinea pigs**
   Allergic rhinitis is predominantly an IgE – mediated inflammation of nasal mucosa and/or cavity, characterized by sneezing, itching, nasal congestion, rhinorrhea, postal nasal drainage and lacrimation of eyes. It is often associated with the loss of smell, taste and induction of cough. All these symptoms are manifested with the results of interaction of resident and infiltrating inflammatory cells along with inflammatory mediators such as cytokines and other neurotransmitters leading to nerve activation, plasma leakage and congestion of venous sinusoids. Various animal models are developed and used for screening and studying etiopathological aspects of allergic rhinitis.

   Guinea pig allergic rhinitis model: Guinea pig is preferred because they mimic human rhinitis and respond to clinical pharmacotherapy. Treat the negative control group with montelukast (100 mg/kg) or sodium chromoglycate 100 mg/ml (20 μl/nostril) and other group with test drug with different doses. After 7 days of parenteral route sensitization, instill topically 60 mg/ml, 20 μl/nostril ovalbumin solutions to animals. A week after the last sensitization, shave the dorsal area of animals by using electric clipper and challenge with intradermal injection of ovalbumin (25 μl of 200 μg/ml). Perform experiments in a room which is free of noise and strong odor, and maintain temperature at 23°C, and relative humidity 55%.

The manifestation of symptoms like edema and redness at the site of injection confirms the successful sensitization. Ovalbumin dose 60 mg/ml (20 μl/nostril) for induction of allergic rhinitis is selected because this dose elicits typical symptoms such as sneezing, nose rubbing, eye lacrimation and difficulty in breathing which are observed for 2 hr (after the local challenge around nostril). (Bahekar et al, 2008).

Scoring symptoms (arbitrarily):
a. Sneezing is generally characterized by an explosive expiration just after a deep inspiration.
b. Nose rubbing is characterized by the external perinasal scratching with either one or both forelimbs of animal.
c. Lacrimation scoring on 3 point scale (i) hazy eyes (+); (ii) lacrimation (++) and (iii) lacrimation with conjunctivitis (+++).
d. Nasal acoustic phenomenon that indicate nasal congestion/obstruction and, assess as impaired inspiration (+), nasal inflammation (++) and severe breathing loss / impairment (+++).
e. Consider nasal secretion (watery fluid) discharged through nostril or trickling on the walls of observation cages during screening as the sign of rhinorrhea.
f. Sacrifice the animals at the end of experiment by following the animal ethics, and dissect nasal cavity from skin, muscle and soft tissues, and preserve in 10% neutral buffered formalin solution until taken up for histopathological examination.

Determine the various biochemical paradigms such as ovalbumin- specific serum IgE, interleukin – 4 (IL-4) and nitric oxide level in nasal lavage and eosinophil peroxide activity in nasal cavity. Such biochemical studies help to understand the probable mode of action of drug and also indicate biochemical alterations occurring during allergic rhinitis. Reference drug, sodium cromoglycate treatment reduce symptoms such as sneezing, rubbing frequencies and prevents the elevation of serum IgE significantly. Both Montelukast and Sodium chromoglycate decrease eosinophil peroxidase activity of nasal cavity significantly. The elevated IL-4 and nitric oxide of nasal lavage are also decreased by the treatment of reference drugs significantly. Thus, the guinea pig allergic rhinitis model is a reliable and reproducible, and used routinely for drug screening program.

7. **Experimentally induced Allergic Conjunctivitis in Guinea Pig**
   Allergic conjunctivitis (AC) is one of the common immune mediated diseases of the eye. The most characteristic of symptoms are ocular itching, hyperemia; edema and nasal secretion that affect the quality of life. Further, the occurrence of allergic conjunctivitis is also rapidly increasing in Indian Population. The AC has two distinct phases: acute phase exhibits the symptoms such as ocular itching, edema associated hyperemia, leads to the cellular filtration into the conjunctiva. The second phase is largely associated with immunoglobulin activated reactions and hence, symptoms persist for longer period.

In allergic conjunctivitis reactions, both H_1 receptor and substance P (belong to tachykinin peptide family) participates and significantly contribute to tissue injury and chronicity.

Experimental methods: Use male 3 week- old guinea pigs and divide into various groups (6 animals/group). Actively sensitize animals by injecting subconjunctivally with 2 μg of ovalbumin (EA) and 2 mg of aluminum hydroxide gel on day zero.

Instill ovalbumin 20 μL of 2.5% EA solution into the conjunctival sac as challenge for the positive control and drug treatment groups on 15, 17 and 19th day or instill PBS into the conjucntival sac of control group. Administer anti-allergic drug such as ketocifen, olopatadine, levocabastine and tranilast 20 μL of each drug to conjucntival sac of the animal 5 min and 15 min prior to the final challenge with EA on 19th day. (Yosuke et al, 2017).

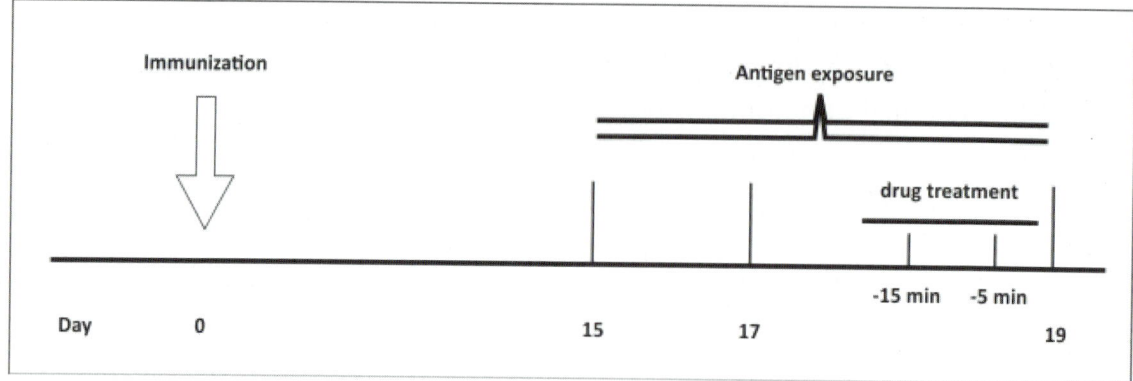

Fig. 8.1: Indicate sensitization process, challenge and drug treatment.

Scratching behavior:

Scratching behavior is counted as an interrupted cluster of rapid hind limb movements that are precisely directed towards eye.

Quantitatively measure the scratching behavior for one hour after the OA challenge on day 15th and 19th day. Count the scratching reactions and quantify on the basis of the number of such responses observed on day 19 and divide by the number of such responses on day 15 for each animal. Consider the mean of scratching reactions of animals for total effect.

Eosinophil assay in epithelial tissues:

Collect conjunctival epithelial cells from upper palpebral conjunctiva with the help of cotton-wool swab 4 hr after OA challenge on 19th day. Spread the swab samples on glass slides, fix and stain with Giemsa staining solutions. Consider the mean of epithelial cell counts of six animals in each group for statistical analysis of the findings. Collect tears 15 minutes after OA challenge on 19th day for determination of the content of histamine and substance P in tears using commercial kits. Quantify histamine and substance P in the samples using UV spectrophotometer at 470 nm.

Increase in histamine and substance P levels are observed in tear after the challenge on 19th day in positive control group, and drug treatment prevent the increase of both histamine and substance P content in tear significantly.

Table 8.1: Drug effects on Allergic Conjunctivitis in Rat Model

Parameters group	Positive Control Group	Drug treated
Behavioral Parameters	Scratching behaviour $\downarrow$	$\downarrow$
Biochemical Parameters in tears	Histamine $\downarrow$ Substance P $\downarrow$	$\downarrow$
Eosinphils of conjunctiva	$\downarrow$	$\downarrow$
Note: Sodium chromoglycate (mast cell stabiliser), Montelukast (Leukotriene receptor blocker), Dexamethasone (broad spectrum activity)		

B. Anti-allergy Drug Screening Methods (*In-Vitro*):

1. **Sensitized isolated guinea pig ileum preparation**

   Sacrifice the sensitized guinea pigs (Sensitize with egg albumin 10 mg/kg, i.p. on day 1, 3, and 9) on the day 14 by observing the necessary animal ethics and remove the ileum, and cut into small segments of 2-3 cm long. Suspend the guinea pig ileum in a organ bath [20 ml capacity containing Tyrode perfusion solution] and aerate with air (95% O_2+CO_2 5%) maintaining organ bath temperature 37°C and connect to force displacement transducer. After setting of isolated ileum preparation, allow tissue for 1 h for attaining equilibrium prior to testing drugs. Record the response of isolated ileum to agonist such as acetylcholine (3.75×10^{-7} M), histamine (2.71×10^{-7} M) and barium chloride (2.05×10^{-3} M) on student physiograph. Repeat the similar responses both in the presence and absence of test compounds or reference drug (aminophylline) at different concentrations. Plot the dose response effect curve with the percentage inhibition of tissue contraction against the different concentrations of agonists in the presence of the test or reference drug. Using the reference drug dose response effect curve, it is possible to determine the potency of the test drug.

2. **Shultz-Dale inhibition test**

   Histamine is one of the major putative mediators in immediate phase of asthma causing airway hyper responsiveness including bronchial inflammation, and demonstrated the involvement of H_1 and H_2 receptors in the experimental asthma model of guinea pig using respiratory smooth muscle and ileum.

Experimental Procedure: Sensitize the guinea pigs with EA (100 mg/kg, i.p.) on 1st, 3rd and 9th day. Administer normal saline 10 ml/kg p.o.) to control group animals and test drug at different doses (p.o. or i.p.) and reference drug [sodium cromoglycate (3 mg/kg, p.o.)] to two different groups of animals for 5 days from 9th day to 13th day during sensitization period. Sacrifice the animals on day 14 (i.e. 24 h after test or reference drug treatment). Separate the ileum segment from each animal and mount on student organ bath and perfuse with Tyrode solution, aerate and maintain the temperature at 37°C. Test the sensitivity of isolated tissue prior to experiments. Add EA (10 μg/ml) and record the tissue response for 90 seconds on a smoked rotating drum (student organ bath). Express the effects in percentage protection against antigen induced anaphylactic reaction (Schultz-Dale reaction).

Further, it is possible to study the direct antigen effect *(ex-in-vivo)* on sensitized ileum with EA 100 mg/kg, i.p. as mentioned above, but without prior treatment of test or reference drug and testing the antigen effect *(ex-in-vivo)* in the presence of test or reference drug at various concentrations (by adding EA 10 μg/ml to the bath). Observe responses of the tissue, and calculate percent protection of contraction of the antigen induced tissue response. Plot a dose response protection curve (responses at different concentrations of test or reference drug to 10 μg/ml of EA). From this curve calculate EC_{50} for test or reference drug in a Shultz –Dale reaction.

3. **Guinea pig tracheal chain preparation**
    Sacrifice the guinea pigs (400-500 g body weight) under ether anesthesia. Separate the skin and muscles of neck, identify, isolate trachea and then remove. Place isolated trachea in a dish containing Kreb's solution immediately. Clean trachea from the surrounding connective tissues until a glistering white cartilaginous surface is observed. The tissue also includes a strip of smooth muscle on the posterior side. Open the trachea by cutting the cartilaginous part vertically in the midline. Subsequently, it also cuts into transverse strips each of which contains a central segment of smooth muscle with cartilage at the ends. Join the strips end to end (depicted in **Fig. 8.2**) and prepare a tracheal chain. Mount the tracheal chain in a student organ bath, and perfuse with Kreb's solution at 37°C and aerate (bubbling with oxygen). Balance the recording isotonic frontal writing lever precisely for a tension of 0.5 g, and allow tracheal chain to relax for 60-90 minutes.

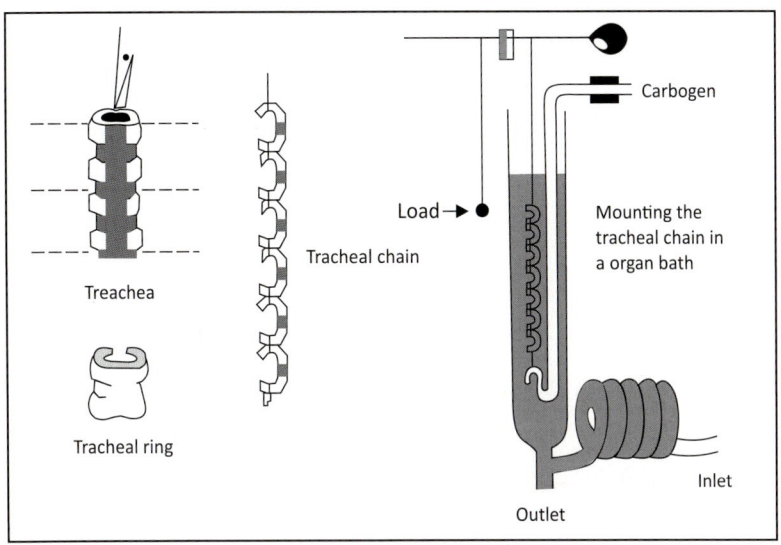

Fig. 8.2: Guinea pig Tracheal Chain Preparation.

Record the tissue responses to drug by maintaining contact period of 90-120 sec and recovery period of 20 minutes. (Castillo, 1948).

- Set up an isolated preparation of guinea pig tracheal chain as described earlier.

- Record the response of graded dose of (agonists), histamine, acetyl choline and 5- hydroxyl tryptamine on a smoked rotating drum (student organ bath).

- Take the response of histamine, acetylcholine and 5-hydroxyl tryptamine on a smooked rotating drum in the presence of test drug (such as plant extracts, synthetic compounds and standard/reference drug).

- Record a dose response curve of agonists by maintaining either varying test compounds concentration or at the optimum effective concentration of test compounds/reference drug in the organ bath. Maintain the test compound minimum contact time 90-120 sec, and then add agonist and observe the tissue response.

4. **Measurement of Histamine Release**

The anti-allergic activity can be evaluated by studying effect of test samples on the induced histamine release from human basophilic cell-line Ku-812. Wash the Ku-812 cell-line and suspend in Tyrode perfusing buffer. Incubate 5.0 Mm calcium ionophore A23187 with test compounds (1.5 mg/ml) and then add to the cell suspension. Incubate the whole mixture at 37°C for 20 minutes. Stop the reaction by maintaining the temperature of reaction mixture at 4°C for 15 minutes. Centrifuge the cell suspension mixture at 10000 g and separate the supernatant and determine histamine content in supernatant by HPLC method using COSMOSIL 5C18-PAQ column. (Junko et al, 2006).

Measure the peak area of the HPLC tracing and then calculate the percentage histamine release by the following formula:

$$\% \text{ histamine release} = \frac{(\text{Test - Negative control})}{\text{Positive control- Negative control}} \times 100$$

C. Anti-asthma drug Screening Methods (*In-Vivo*)

Generally rodents do not spontaneously develop airway hyper responsiveness to allergic airway inflammation; hence it is necessary to induce artificial asthma like reaction in the airways.

1. Primary allergic challenge model:

This model is used widely to demonstrate the underlying events in immunologic and inflammatory responses in airways. This involves both basic phase of sensitization as well as the challenge phase. The primary allergic challenge models are of short term duration and always show high degree of reproducibility.

Airway inflammation and airway hyper-reactivity are known to resolve with few weeks after final allergen inhalation. Therefore, it is considered as an acute allergic pulmonary inflammation. In this model, a wide range of useful cellular and molecular model systems are used (such as anti-cytokine mediator antagonist's approaches, platelet activating factor, Very Late Antigen-4 (VLA-4), and specific enzyme inhibitors). However, afore mentioned systems are only useful in acute challenge animal models, and need to be demonstrated clinically in patients. IL-5 is an important mediator and appears to play a key role in allergen induced inflammatory response and also development of airway hyper reactivity. Hence, this is necessary to establish clinically in asthmatic patients.

Experimental Procedure: Select and divide randomly female BALB/c mice, aged 6-8 weeks into different groups (6/group), and administer the following treatments: (a) sham-sensitization plus challenge with PBS (i.p.); (b) sensitization plus challenge with OVA (i.p.); (c) sensitization with OVA (i.p.) plus challenge with OVA (aerosol), and test drug or reference drug [Dexamethasone (3 mg/kg, p.o.) and Montelukast (50 mg/kg, p.o.)].

Sensitize the mice by intraperitoneal injection of 20 μg OVA emulsified in 2 mg aluminum hydroxide in 100 μL PBS buffer (pH 7.4), on days 0 and 14.

Challenge the each mouse through the airway with OVA (1%, w/v, in PBS) for 20 min using an ultrasonic nebulizer (NE-U12; Omron Corp., Tokyo, Japan) on days 28, 29, and 30 after initial sensitization.

Administer test and reference drug daily (p.o./i.p.) to mice from days 18-30.

Forty eight hours after the last challenge (i.e. day 32) sacrifice the mice to assess suppressive effects of test and reference drug on airway hyper responsiveness reactions. (Lee et al, 2011).

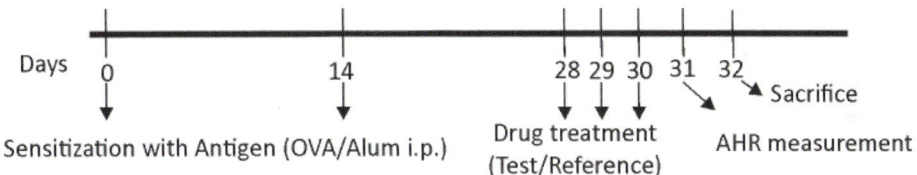

Days 0   14   28 29 30 31 32   Sacrifice

Sensitization with Antigen (OVA/Alum i.p.)   Drug treatment (Test/Reference)   AHR measurement

Fig. 8.3: **Mouse model of airway inflammation and treatment with test / reference drug.**

Measurement of airway hyper responsiveness (AHR):

Assess AHR in conscious and unrestrained mice by whole body plethysmography (OCP3000 instrument; Allmedicus, Seoul, Korea) 24 h after the final aerosol challenge.

Each mouse was placed in a plastic chamber and exposed to aerosolized PBS, followed by aerosols containing increasing concentrations of methacholine (6.25, 12.5 and 25 mg/mL; Sigma) in PBS, for 3 min at each exposure level.

Place each mouse in a plastic chamber and expose to aerosolized PBS, then again exposé the each mouse for 3 min at each exposure level to aerosols containing increasing concentrations of methacholine (6.25, 12.5 and 25 mg/mL;) in PBS.

Record the bronchoconstriction of each mouse for an additional 5 min after each methacholine exposure. Observe and measure the highest enhanced pause (Penh) value during each methacholine challenge and calculate a proportion of the basal enhanced pause (Penh) value in response to PBS challenge.

Eosinophil and Differential leukocytes numbers in Bronchoalveolar fluid (BALF):

Sacrifice the mice, 48 h after the last challenge (i.e. on day 32) or just before death of animal, lavage the tracheobronchial tree with 2 ml of normal saline. Collect the fluid by tracheal cannulation and centrifuge at 2000 rpm for 10 minutes at 4°C. Discard the supernatant and resuspend pellet in 0.5 ml normal saline and prepare its thin film (0.05 ml pellet normal saline solution) and fix with methyl alcohol for 5 minutes and dry. Then stain the film with Friedel solution A & B, and for differential leukocyte count, stain the film with Geimsa stain. Determine the total number of eosinphils and leucocytes in 0.05 ml fluid under the microscope with 450 × magnification.

Histopathology of Lung tissue

After the separation of BALF, fix the lung tissue in 10% (v/v) neutral buffered formalin for 24 h. Embed the tissues in paraffin, cut into sections of 4 μm thickness, stain with H & E solution (hematoxylin, Sigma MHS-16, and eosin, Sigma HT110-1-32) and with periodic acid Schiff (PAS) stain (IMEB Inc., San Marcos, CA), to measure mucus production. Mount the tissues subsequently and covered slip using Dako-mounting medium (Dakocytomation, Denmark, CA). Score the degree of airway inflammatory cell infiltration in a double-blind manner by independent investigators. Quantify the Goblet-cell hyperplasia in airway epithelium by following a five-point system: 0, no goblet cells; 1, <25% of epithelium; 2, 25–50% of epithelium; 3, 50–75% of epithelium; 4, >75% of epithelium. Analyze five airway sections randomly distributed through the left lung for each mouse and calculate average scores. Perform quantitative analysis of mucus production by using an image analyzer (Leica Microsystems Imaging Solutions Ltd., Cambridge, UK).

2. **Secondary Allergen Challenge Model:**

The secondary allergen experimental model is developed to simulate conditions of allergen asthma with allergen re-challange of animals after sensitization and primary allergen challenge. In this experiment, preferably BALB/c mice are used. Exposure of mice to secondary challenge after 2-6 weeks following primary exposure (challenge) because by this time generally airway eosinophilia and air way hyper activity is get resolved and attains normal levels. This simulation is very much similar to that of guinea pig model of bronchial asthma induced with egg-albumin and trypsin.

Experimental Procedure: Select and divide randomly guinea pigs into different groups (6/group). Exposure of guinea pigs once daily to aerosol of trypsin (1 mg/ml, 1 ml/min) for 5 minutes and allow to rest for 2 hours, and there after subject them to egg – albumin (1% solution, 1 ml/min) aerosol exposure for 10 minutes. Repeat same procedure for 10 days. Subsequently, stop egg- albumin aerosol but continue trypsin exposure for 21st day. On the 22nd day test guinea pigs for different pulmonary function and parameters described above for confirming the development of bronchial asthma.

After confirming of asthma, expose guinea pigs of normal control group to aerosol of saline for 5 minutes daily. Expose guinea pigs of positive control group to trypsin and egg albumin without any drug treatment. Daily administer dexamethasone (5 mg/kg, p.o.) and test drug from day 22-35 to guinea pigs of respective groups. Challenge guinea pigs with only egg albumin on day 35, after 2 h of the last dose of treatment. Determine the various parameters related to pulmonary function such as PO_2, tidal volume, respiratory rate, serum bicarbonate on day 1 (baseline) prior to any exposure, on day 21 (after trypsin exposure), and on day 35 (after treatment) for each animal. In addition to above parameters, on day 35, measure eosinophil count in BALF and perform histopathology of lung tissue.

In this modified method rats and mice can also be used in place of guinea-pigs. In this procedure trypsin can be replaced by adenosine, as this is also known to participate as one of the putative mediator in the development of bronchial asthma. (Patel and Chorawala, 2011, Shah et al, 2017).

3. **Chronic Allergen Challenge Models**

A chronic allergen challenge mice model is very much similar and closely resembles (mimic) to human asthma. In this model, BALB/c mice are preferred. This method involves exposure of mice to increasing number of allergen over many weeks (10-15 weeks). The allergens such as grass pollen and antigen like ovalbumin are used. The major drawback of this method is long term exposure generally leads to the development of tolerance, and a steady decrease in airway hyper responsiveness and eosinophilia. The chronic model largely reproduces the characteristic symptoms of asthma such as goblet cell metaplasia, epithelial hypertrophy, sub epithelial fibrosis and mild smooth muscle hyperplasia.

Evaluation parameters for *in-vivo* models

i) Partial pressure of oxygen (PO_2):

In this, measurement of arterial O_2 tension (PO_2) is perfomed using pulse oxymeter, and detection of oxygen saturation of hemoglobin by spectrophotometer (based on Beer – Lambart Law) which is directly proportional to concentration of solute to the intensity of light transmission in solution.

ii) Partial pressure of carbon dioxide (PCO_2):

PCO_2 measurement is performed by Capnometer. The arterial CO_2 tension (PCO_2) explains the ratio between metabolism and effective volume of the breathing which is the indication of alveolar ventilation. The ratio of the arterial PCO_2 α volume of CO_2 produced / Alveolar ventilation. The mentioned ratio is between the volume of CO_2 production and alveolar ventilation and hence, the CO_2 remains relatively constant in normal physiological condition (in healthy person) over a wide range of CO_2 production. If alveolar ventilation is inadequate the CO_2 level increases, and if alveolar ventilation is excessive the level of PCO_2 falls.

iii) Serum bicarbonate level:

Collect 3 ml blood from retro orbital plexus under light ether anesthesia following one hour exposure to allergen. Separate serum by minimum exposure to air and store in a sealed tube until bicarbonate is assayed.

iv) Measurement of tidal volume

Tidal volume is the volume of air inspired or expired per breath during normal breath. The tidal volume is measured with the help of "Respiratory Volume Transducer" that is used with "Strain Gauge Coupler" and student physiograph. On well calibrated physiograph (normally with the help of 0.02 and 0.1 cc volume air supplier) the tidal volume is measured in terms of height of response. Subsequently the height is converted to volume.

v) Measurement of respiratory rate:

Measure respiratory rate and express as breath/minute. Record the respiratory waves for the tidal volume and count for a period of one minute. Express the results as breath/minute.

vi) Air flow rate measurement:

It is defined as a volume of air inspired or expired per unit time during normal breathing (ml/min). It is calculated as Airflow rate = Respiratory rate

vii) Superoxide dismutase (SOD) level measurement:

SOD is an endogenous enzyme and has the ability to inhibit the auto-oxidation of epinephrine to adrenochrome at pH 10.2. Such inhibition is measured calorimetrically at 480 nm. Enhanced oxidative stress and reduced SOD activity in asthmatic airway is directly correlated with airflow limitation and hyperactivity.

Similarly, reduced glutathione plays a critical role in balancing intracellular oxidation – reduction event in normal physiological condition. Hence, determination of glutathione status can serve an important index in oxidative stress.

viii) Eosinophil and differential leukocytes numbers in bronchoalveolar fluid (BALF):

Sacrifice the animals or just before death of animal, lavage the tracheobronchial tree with 2 ml of normal saline. Collect the fluid by tracheal cannulation and centrifuge at 2000 rpm for 10 minutes at 4°C. Discard the supernatant and resuspend pellet in 0.5 ml normal saline and prepare its thin film (0.05 ml pellet normal saline solution) and fix with methyl alcohol for 5 minutes and dry. Then stain the film with

Friedel solution A & B, and for differential leukocyte count, stain the film with Geimsa stain. Determine the total number of eosinphils and leucocytes in 0.05 ml fluid under the microscope with 450 × magnification.

ix) Forced expiratory volume (FEV1), Forced Vital Capacity (FVC) and Peak Expiratory Flow rate (PEFR):
The most sensitive test for determining abnormalities in airway function is the forced expiratory volume. The FEV1 is the measure of the forced expiratory volume in the first second of exhalation.

Forced vital capacity is the measurement of the maximum volume of air exhalation with maximum effort after maximum inspiration. Express FEV1 as a percentage of the total volume of air inhalation and calculate the ratio as FEV1/FVC.

The peak flow meter determines peak expiratory flow rate, i.e. the maximum flow rate that can be forced during expiration. The PEFR is an useful index for assessing the improvement or deterioration during the disease as well as the effectiveness after drug treatment.

Experimental procedure: Briefly, animals are anaesthetized with ketamine (80 mg/kg, i.p.) and then trachea is punctured using surgical blade without disturbing the other vasculature to avoid the blood loss. Subsequently, angiocatheter of number 26 is passing via the tracheal puncture and other end is connected to the respiratory pod of PowerLab 26T instrument (AD Instruments Pty Ltd., Australia). Using the LabTutor 4 Suit Software of the above instrument, the following parameters are measured:
• Time of inspiration (sec)
• Time of expiration (sec)
• Breathing frequency (number of breaths/min)
• Forced expiratory volume (FEV1)
• Forced Vital Capacity (FVC)
• Peak Expiratory Flow rate (PEFR)

The documented publication suggest that dexamethasone at lower doses (2-5 mg/kg) and other clinically effective anti-asthmatic drugs improve significantly, the impaired above mentioned pulmonary function related parameters.

References:

1. Bahekar, P.C., Shah, J.H., Ayer, U.B., Mandhane, S.N., Thennati, R., 2008. Validation of guinea pig model of allergic rhinitis by oral and topical drugs. Int Immunopharmacol, 8, 1540–51.

2. Bhargava, K.P., Singh, N., 1981. Anti-stress activity of Ocimum sanctum Linn. Indian J Med Res 73, 443-451.

3. Castillo, J.C., 1948. The tracheal chain; the anaphylactic guinea pig trachea and its response to antihistamine and bronchodilator drugs. J Pharmacol Exp Ther, 94, 412-415.

4. Hachisuka, H., Kusuhara, M., Higuchi, M., Okubo, K., Sasai, Y., 1988. Purification of rat mast cells with percoll density centrifugation. Archives of Dermatology Research 280, 358–362.

5. Han, S.J., Bae, E.A., Trinh, H.T., Yang, J.H., Youn, U.J., Bae, K.H., Kim, D.H., 2007. Magnolol and honokiol: inhibitors against mouse passive cutaneous anaphylaxis reaction and scratching behaviors. Biol. Pharm. Bull. 30, 2201-2203.

6. Koyama, J., Morita, I., Kobayashi, N., Hirai, K., Simamura, E., Nobukawa, T., Kadota, S., 2006. Antiallergic activity of aqueous extracts and constituents of Taxus yunnanensis. Biol Pharm Bull. 29, 2310-2312.

7. Lee, M.Y., Seo, C.S., Lee, J.A., Lee, N.H., Kim, J.H., Ha, H., Zheng, M.S., Son, J.K., Shin, H.K., 2011. Anti-asthmatic effects of Angelica dahurica against ovalbumin-induced airway inflammation via upregulation of heme oxygenase-1. Food Chem Toxicol, 49, 829-37.

8. Mitra, S.K., Gopumadhavan, S., Venkataranganna, M.V., Anturlikar, S.D., 1999. Anti-asthmatic and anti-anaphylactic effect of E-721B, a herbal formulation. Indian J. Pharmacol. 31, 133-137.

9. Naik, S.R., Hule, A., 2009. Evaluation of immunomodulatory activity of an extract of andographolides from Andographis paniculata. Planta Med, 75, 785-91.

10. Patel, K.N., and Chorawala, M.R., 2011. Animal models of Asthma. J. Pharma Research and Opinion (JPRO), 1, 139-147.

11. Shah, J.H., Anand, I.H., Shah, K.K., 2017. Effect of Boerhaavia diffusa on Experimental Induced Model of Asthma in Mice. Ijppr.Human, 10, 139-148.

12. Taur, D.J., and Patil, R.Y., 2012. Effect of Abrus precatorius leaves on milk induced leukocytosis and eosinophilia in the management of asthma. Asian Pacific Journal of Tropical Biomedicine, S40-S42.

13. Yosuke, N., Mikako, O., Mokoto, T., 2017. Model for studying anti-allergic drugs for allergic conjunctivitis in animals. Open Med, 12, 231-238.

INTRODUCTION

Diuretics are the drugs that inhibit the reabsorption of water from the tubules and thereby increase the volume of the urine. As the diuretics increase the rate of urination, they provide means for forced diuresis. Different types of diuretics include thiazide diuretics, loop diuretics, potassium sparing diuretics, carbonic anhydrase inhibitors, osmotic agents, xanthenes, vasopressin type 2 receptors antagonists and arginine vasopressin V_2 receptor antagonists.

Three main steps of urine formation include glomerular filtration, tubular reabsorption and tubular secretion. As shown in **Fig. 9.1**, most of the diuretics act on tubule portion of the nephrone and thereby inhibits reabsorption of sodium and other electrolytes.

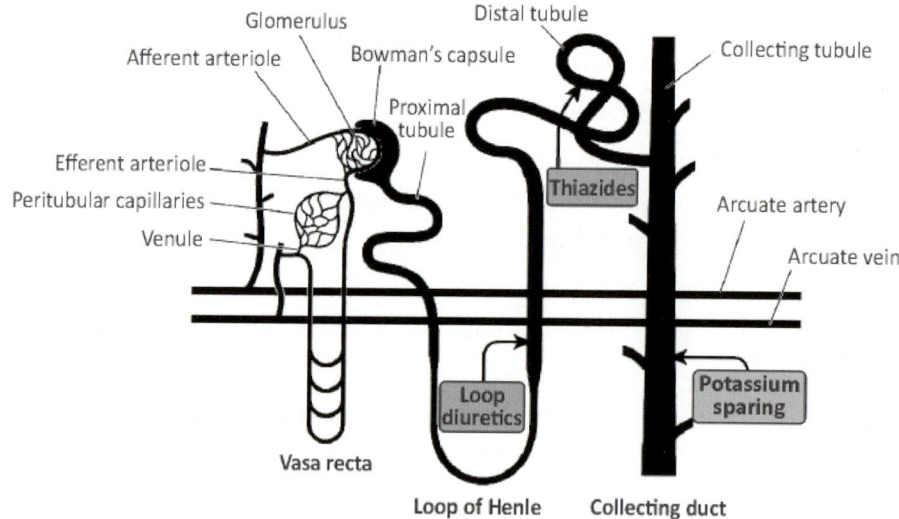

Fig. 9.1: Sites of action of diuretics.

Proximal tubule is the site responsible for tubular reabsorption and secretion. It is involved in reabsorption of filtered glucose, amino acids, filtered sodium bicarbonate and sodium chloride. It is the site of secretion of drugs like penicillin, thiazide diuretics and loop diuretics.

Loop of Henle is an important site for reabsorption of filtered sodium chloride through Na^+, K^+, $2Cl^-$ Symporter and also contributes in formation of concentrated urine by transporting the sodium chloride to the surrounding interstitium.

Early portion of distal tubule is responsible for reabsorption of filtered sodium chloride through Na^+, Cl^- symporter. Collecting duct is responsible for adjustment of final composition and volume of urine through the actions of aldosterone and antidiuretic hormone. Aldosterone, a mineralocorticoid promotes reabsorption of sodium whereas antidiuretic hormone promotes reabsorption of water from the collecting duct.

Each class of diuretics acts on different site of tubular portion to achieve diuretic effect. Diuretics like thiazides act on early portion of distal tubule whereas loop diuretics act on thick ascending limb of loop of Henle. Potassium sparing diuretics act on collecting tubule and carbonic anhydrase inhibitors act on proximal tubule.

Table 9.1: Sites of action and mechanism of action of diuretics

Class of Diuretics	Site of action	Examples	Mechanism of action
Thiazide diuretics	Distal tubule	Hydrochor-thiazide, Chlorthiazide Indapamide	Inhibit reabsorption of Na^+ and Cl^- by inhibiting Na^+, Cl^- symporter in early portion of distal tubule
Loop diuretics	Loop of Henle	Furosemide Ethacrynic acid Bumetanide Torsemide	Inhibit reabsorption of Na^+ by inhibiting membrane bound Na^+, K^+, $2Cl^-$ symporter
Potassium sparing diuretics	Collecting tubule	Amiloride Spironolactone	Amiloride inhibit reabsorption of Na^+ by blocking the exchange of sodium for potassium in

Class of Diuretics	Site of action	Examples	Mechanism of action
			collecting tubule through epithelial sodium channels whereas spironolactone inhibits action of aldosterone
Carbonic anhydrase inhibitors	Proximal tubule	Acetazolamide Dorzolamide	Inhibit reabsorption of sodium bicarbonate due to inhibition of enzyme carbonic anhydrase
Osmotic agents	Proximal tubule, descending loop, collecting duct	Mannitol Urea	Increase in urine output via osmosis
Xanthenes diuretics	Tubule, Glomerulus	Theophylline Theobromine	Rapidly increases urinary concentration of sodium and chloride with a concomitant increase in rate of their excretion, increases glomerular filtration rate that accounts for a part of the diuretic action
Vasopressin type 2 (V_2) receptors antagonists	Collecting tubule	Conivaptan Tolvaptan Lixivaptan Satavaptan	Inhibits V_2 receptors in the collecting duct, alters the expression of aquaporin channels thereby producing aquaresis
Arginine vasopressin (AVP) V_2 receptor antagonists	Tubule	Amphotericin B Lithium citrate	Inhibits the arginine vasopressin V_2 receptor mediated renal water reabsorption, inhibits Na^+ reabsorption

Thiazide diuretics inhibit Na^+, Cl^- symporter in early portion of distal tubule and inhibit reabsorption of Na^+ and Cl^- from the tubular fluid. This causes increase in excretion of both sodium and chloride in the urine so that water is excreted with them. Loop diuretics inhibit Na^+, K^+, $2Cl^-$ symporter in ascending limb of loop of Henle thereby exerting a strong natriuretic effect. Potassium sparing diuretics block the exchange of sodium for potassium at collecting tubule resulting in excretion of sodium with comparatively little loss of potassium.

Potassium sparing diuretics like amiloride block the exchange of sodium for potassium in collecting tubule and enhance the excretion of sodium with comparatively little loss of potassium whereas spironolactone inhibits Na^+ reabsortion by inhibiting action of aldosterone. Carbonic anhydrase inhibitors inhibit reabsorption of sodium bicarbonate from the proximal tubule due to inhibition of enzyme carbonic anhydrase.

Hyponatremia is one of the commonly observed electrolyte abnormality. Vasopressin receptor antagonists are newly introduced group of non-peptide drugs that are used in hyponatremia. They produce aquaresis by their action on vasopressin type 2 (V_2) receptors in the collecting duct and thus increase solute free water excretion. They are used as an alternative to fluid restriction in euvolemic and hypervolemic hyponatremic patients. Arginine vasopressin V_2 receptor antagonists inhibit the arginine vasopressin V_2 receptor mediated renal water reabsorption. It also inhibits Na^+ reabsorption.

Abnormalities in fluid volume and electrolyte composition are common and important clinical problems. Drugs that block the transport functions of the renal tubules therefore become valuable clinical tools in the treatment of these disorders. There are several diseases like congestive heart failure, liver disease and kidney disease which cause the accumulation of fluid within the various tissues of the body. Diuretics are the drugs that increase the formation of urine and thus remove excess extra-cellular water from the edematous tissue and thereby play a role in managing these conditions.

Diuretics are class of drugs that are mainly used to promote increased urinary sodium and urine volume output, which leads to a reduction in the volume of circulating blood, thus decrease blood pressure. Hypertension is a predisposing factor for stroke, coronary heart disease, peripheral arterial disorders, heart failure and renal failure.

Procedure:

Wistar rats weighing 150-200 g are randomly divided into groups of three, each group comprising 6 rats. The groups are labeled as negative control group, positive control group and test drug group. Prior to the commencement of the actual experiment, the rats are placed in an individual metabolic cage 24 hrs for adaptation and then fasted overnight with free access to water. The animals are pre-treated with physiological saline (0.9% NaCl) at an oral dose of 10 ml/kg to impose a uniform water and salt load.

Negative control group is treated with the vehicle used for reconstitution (distilled water orally, 10 ml/kg) whereas positive control group is treated with standard drug (hydrochlorthiazide orally, 10 mg/kg). Test drug is administered to the test drug group in prescribed dosage with prescribed route of administration.

For studying acute diuretic activity, respective groups received single dose of respective treatment. Rats are placed individually in metabolic cages having a wire mesh bottom and a funnel for collecting the urine as shown in **Fig. 9.2**. The urine is collected at 1h, 2h, 3h, 4h and 5h after drug treatment.

The method is slightly modified for estimation of chronic diuretic activity where respective groups received respective treatment for 28 days at a predetermined

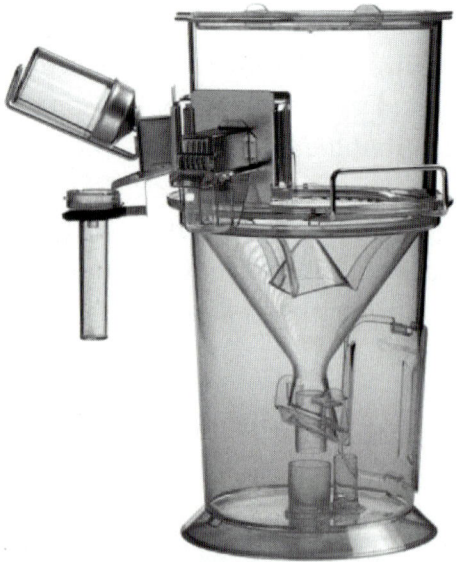

Fig. 9.2: Metabolic cage.

time. Rats are individually placed in metabolic cages on 1st, 7th, 14th, 21st and 28th day for collecting the urine. The urine is collected in each of the collecting flasks and measured using a graduated measuring cylinder. Rats are not allowed food and water during the experimental period.

Evaluation:

Cumulative urine volume is measured. Urine volume of all experimental groups is compared using appropriate statistical methods. Ratio of total urinary output in test group to total urinary output in the control group is calculated to determine the urinary excretion. The ratio of urinary excretion in test group to urinary excretion in the control group is calculated to determine the diuretic action of the test drug. Diuretic activity is assessed by comparing the diuretic action of test group to that of the standard group.

Observation Table

Table 9.2: Study of acute diuretic activity of test drug:

Experimental Groups	Treatment	Dose	Urine volume (ml)				
Vehicle Control	Normal saline	10 ml/kg, oral	1 hr	2 hr	3 hr	4 hr	5 hr
Positive control	Hydrochlo-rthiazide	10 mg/kg, oral					
Test drug group	Drug sample to be tested	Prescribed dose					

Table 9.3: Study of chronic diuretic activity of test drug:

Experimental Groups	Treatment	Dose	Urine volume (ml) (Day)				
			1	7	14	21	28
Control	Distilled water	10 ml/kg, oral					
Positive control	Hydrochlo-rthiazide	10 mg/kg, oral					
Test drug group	Drug sample to be tested	Prescribed dose					

Study of saluretic effect, natriuretic effect and carbonic anhydrase inhibitory activity of test sample

Theory:

Diuresis has two components namely increase in urine volume and a net loss of solutes in the urine. These processes result from suppression of renal tubular reabsorption of water and electrolytes into the blood stream. Both urine volume and electrolyte concentrations are measured to evaluate the saluretic effect, natriuretic effect and carbonic anhydrase inhibitory activity of test sample.

Procedure:

Wistar rats weighing 150-200 g are randomly divided into groups of three, each group comprising 6 rats. The groups are labeled as negative control group, positive control group and test drug group. Prior to the commencement of the actual experiment, the rats are placed in an individual metabolic cage 24 hrs for adaptation and then fasted overnight with free access to water. The animals are pre-treated with physiological saline (0.9% NaCl) at an oral dose of 10 ml/kg to impose a uniform water and salt load.

Negative control group is treated with the vehicle used for reconstitution (distilled water orally, 10 ml/kg) whereas positive control group is treated with standard drugs (furosemide orally, 25 mg/kg). Test drug is administered to the test drug group in prescribed dosage with prescribed route of administration.

Rats are placed individually in metabolic cages having a wire mesh bottom and a funnel for collecting the urine. The urine is collected at the end of 5 h after dosing. Urine pH is measured with a standard pH meter. Sodium content of the urine is measured by flame photometry whereas chloride content is measured by potentiometric titration. Urinary calcium, magnessium, urea, creatinine, glucose and total proteins are measured by automated biochemistry analyzer.

The magnitude of Na^+, K^+ and Cl^- excretion is determined as a parameter for saluretic activity. Saliuretic index is calculated as the ratio of electrolyte in the urine of test group to the concentration of electrolyte in the urine of positive control group.

The ratio Na^+/K^+ is calculated as an indicator for natriuretic activity. Values greater than 2.0 indicate a favorable natriuretic effect, while ratios greater than 10.0 indicate a potassium-sparing effect.

The ratio Cl^-/Na^++K^+ is calculated as carbonic anhydrase index and is an indicator of carbonic anhydrase inhibitory activity.

Observation Table:

Table 9.4: Effect of test sample on urinary electrolytes and saluretic index

Experimental Groups	Treatment	Dose	Urinary Electrolyte Concentration (mmol/lt)			Saluretic index		
			Na^+	K^+	Cl^-	Na^+	K^+	Cl^-
Control	Distilled water	10 ml/kg, oral						
Positive control	Furosemide	25 mg/kg, oral						
Test drug	Drug sample to be tested	Prescribed dose						

Table 9.5: Effect of test sample on natriuresis and carbonic anhydrase (CA) inhibition

Experimental Groups	Treatment	Dose	Natriuretic activity	CA inhibition
			Na^+/K^+	Cl^-/Na^++K^+
Control	Distilled water	10 ml/kg, oral		
Positive control	Furosemide	25 mg/kg, oral		
Test drug	Drug sample to be tested	Prescribed dose		

References:

1. Kau, S.T., Keddie, J.R., Andrews, D., 1984. A method for screening diuretic agents in the rat. J. Pharmacol. Methods 11, 67–75.

2. Mukherjee, P.K. 2002. Evaluation of diuretic agents In: Quality Control of Herbal Drugs Business Horizons, New Delhi. Publishers Ltd., India, p. 564.

3. Yu, C.H., Tang, W.Z., Penga, C., Suna, T., Liuc, B., Li, M., et al., 2012. Diuretic, antiinflammatory, and analgesic activities of the ethanol extract from Cynoglossum lanceolatum. J. Ethnopharmacol. 139, 149–154.

4. Nedi, T., Mekonnena, N., Urga, K., 2004. Diuretic effect of the crude extracts of Carissa edulis in rats. J. Ethnopharmacol. 95 (1), 57–61.

5. Peri A. 2013. Clinical review: the use of vaptans in clinical endocrinology J Clin Endocrinol Metab. 98(4), 1321-32.

6. Beharu, W., Teshome, N., Workineh, S., Mekonnen S. 2017. Evaluation of the diuretic activity of the aqueous and 80% methanol extracts of the root of Euclea divinorum Hiern (Ebenaceae) in Sprague Dawley rats. Journal of Ethnopharmacol. 202, 114–121.

7. Amuthana, A., Chogtub, B., Bairyb, K.L., Prakash, S.M., 2002. Evaluation of diuretic activity of Amaranthus spinosus Linn. aqueous extract in Wistar rats. J. Ethnopharmacol. 140, 424–427.

INTRODUCTION TO OXIDATIVE STRESS

Free radicals are formed when oxygen interacts with certain molecules (Mazumdar et al. 2012). Free radicals are produced as a consequence of normal biochemical reactions in the body (Surveswaran et al. 2007). They are atoms or groups of atoms which contain at least one unpaired electron in their orbital. A free radical is also treated as unstable form of any atom or molecule and could be generated in the body in many distinct ways like (a) breaking of covalent bonds by hemolytic way (b) losing an electron (c) gaining an electron. Free radicals constitute of hydroxyl ($OH\bullet$), superoxide ($O_2\bullet^-$), nitric oxide ($NO\bullet$), nitrogen dioxide ($NO_2\bullet$), peroxyl ($ROO\bullet$) and lipid peroxyl ($LOO\bullet$). Furthermore, oxidants like hydrogen peroxide (H_2O_2), ozone (O_3), singlet oxygen ($1O_2$), hypochlorous acid ($HOCl$), nitrous acid (HNO_2), peroxynitrite ($ONOO^-$), dinitrogen trioxide (N_2O_3) and lipid peroxide ($LOOH$), although not being free radicals, yet can freely lead to free radical reactions in living beings. Free radicals are produced inside the body in massive varieties. In the midst of all the free radicals, reactive oxygen species (ROS) and reactive nitrogen species (RNS) are the prominent ones. ROS and RNS are generated from either endogenous or exogenous sources (Mazumdar et al. 2012). Reactive oxygen species (ROS) have a cogent effect on the internal as well as external body environment of human beings (Selvakumar et al. 2011). ROS and RNS are well known for playing a bifold role as both detrimental and constructive species, as they can be either harmful or beneficial to living systems. At low and moderate conditions ROS and RNS play crucial role in maintaining normal physiological functions of the body chiefly in the immune system, maturation process of cell structures, cell signaling mechanisms (Mazumdar et al. 2012). ROS such as superoxide (O_2^-), hydroxyl ($OH\bullet$) and hydrogen peroxide (H_2O_2) are either arisen normally during metabolism or are devised ardently by the immune cells to neutralize the foreign bodies. The ROS damages crucial proteins, DNA and lipids and becomes the origin of various human diseases such as atherosclerosis, cancer, liver injury, cardiovascular disease, neurodegenerative disorders and rheumatism as a consequence of 'Oxidative Stress'. Thus, the harmful effect of free radicals causing probable biological damage is termed oxidative stress and nitrosative stress. Exogenous ROS/RNS are results of air and water pollution, cigarette smoke, alcohol, heavy or transition metals (Cd, Hg, Pb, Fe, As), certain drugs (cyclosporine, tacrolimus, gentamycin, bleomycin), industrial solvents, cooking (smoked meat, used oil, fat) and radiation. Thus, oxidative stress is essentially produced due to the imbalance between the formation of free radicals and antioxidants in the body. It is also presently proposed as the mechanism underpinning diabetes and diabetes induced complications (Mazumdar et al. 2012).

INTRODUCTION TO ANTIOXIDANTS

In spite of the body's defense mechanism in the form of enzymes & antioxidant nutrients which restrain the damaging properties of reactive oxygen species, unceasing exposure to chemicals and contaminants may raise the amount of free radicals in the body over its capacity to manage and thus, cause irreversible oxidative damage. Hence, there arises the need of antioxidants which are substances that when present at low concentrations, compared to those of the oxidizable substrate significantly delay or inhibit the oxidation of the substrate (Selvakumar et al. 2011). Thus, antioxidants are defined as the defense system of the body against free radicals. Antioxidants interact with free radicals and block them before integral molecules are damaged. Antioxidants are produced within the body. At the same time, they can also be derived from the food we eat like fruits, vegetables, seeds, nuts, meats and oil (Mazumdar et al. 2012).

IMPORTANCE OF ANTIOXIDANTS

Antioxidants with free radical scavenging potential may be pertinent in the prevention and therapeutics of diseases where free radicals are involved. World health organization has approved the use of natural antioxidants which can delay or impede the lipids or other molecules oxidation by inhibiting the genesis or propagation of oxidative chain reactions. The most crucial role of antioxidants is to quench free radical-mediated oxidation by impeding the formation of free radicals by scavenging radicals. Radical scavenging action relies on both the reactivity and concentration of the antioxidant. Hence, the redox properties of antioxidants play a crucial role in absorbing and neutralizing free radicals, quenching singlet and triplet oxygen, or decomposing peroxides. However, in this process, the antioxidants themselves become oxidized. This drives the perpetual demand of antioxidants to replenish them. The antioxidants work mechanistically with two prime functions. They act as the giver of the hydrogen atom which is the first and the main function. The second function is secondary which is preventive in nature wherein antioxidants reduce the rate of auto-oxidation with a variety of mechanisms beyond the auto-oxidation mechanism of chain termination by radical conversion of lipids to form more stable i.e. by scavenging initiating radicals (Selvakumar et al. 2011). Enzymes such as superoxide dismutase, catalase and glutathione peroxidase present in the human body provide innate defense mechanisms to antagonise free radicals. Literature survey proposes the use of vitamin C, vitamin E, selenium, β-carotene, lycopene, lutein and other carotenoids as supplementary antioxidants. Additionally, plant secondary metabolites such as flavonoids and terpenoids have exhibited a crucial role in the defense against free radicals. Ayurvedic preparations from various plant extracts, known as Rasayanas are recognized to contain potent antioxidants and are used as rejuvenators or nutritional supplements. In case of phenolic acids and flavonoids the antioxidant properties are attributed to their redox properties, ability to chelate metals and quenching of singlet oxygen (Surveswaran et al. 2007).

ANTIOXIDANT SCREENING METHODS AND ITS SIGNIFICANCE

In many fields antioxidant research has become functioning to an enormous extent (Selvakumar et al. 2011). Antioxidant capacities can be evaluated by 2,2'-azinobis-3-ethylbenzothiazoline-6-sulfonic acid (ABTS), 1,1-diphenyl-2-picrylhydrazyl (DPPH), ferric reducing antioxidant power (FRAP) assays (Surveswaran et al. 2007). Choosing a competent assay is demanding to examine the antioxidant activity of biological samples (Selvakumar et al. 2011). Antioxidant screening techniques can give clues to the exploration of valuable antioxidant drugs (Surveswaran et al. 2007). Literature survey indicated that Auddy et al. (2003) used the ABTS method and lipid peroxidation assay to evaluate the antioxidant potential of three species, *Sida cordifolia*, *Evolvulus alsinoides*, and *Cyanodon dactylon*, which are used in the treatment of neurodegenerative disorders. However, the above mentioned study included only two assay methods. A comparative, multi-method screening of antioxidant activity is desired to provide a better perception of their relative importance as natural antioxidants. Methods such as ABTS, oxygen radical absorbance capacity (ORAC), DPPH, FRAP have been used in the past to access the total antioxidant capacity (Surveswaran et al. 2007). However, for systematic evaluation of drugs for their antioxidant potential it is vital to carry out more than one of the following antioxidant assays. Hence, this chapter aims to be extensive to cover antioxidant assays which have few significance and applications. It summarizes the adaptability of antioxidants against the free radicals, their mechanism of action and the chemical principles of most of the antioxidant assays.

VARIOUS ANTIOXIDANT TESTS

A. Qualitative antioxidant assays

- DPPH (1,1-Diphenyl-2-picryl-hydrazyl) radical scavenging assay
- ABTS (2,2'-azino-bis3-ethylbenzthiazoline-6-sulfonic) radical scavenging assay
- Nitric oxide scavenging assay
- Hydroxyl radical scavenging assay
- Superoxide radical scavenging activity assay
- Hydrogen peroxide scavenging activity assay
- ORAC (Oxygen radical absorbance capacity) assay
- β-Carotene/Linoleic assay
- Reducing power assay
- Ferric reducing antioxidant power assay
- Phosphomolybdenum assay
- Bovine serum albumin oxidative damage assay
- Lipid peroxidation assay
- Metal ion chelation assay
  - Cupric ions chelation assay
  - Ferrous ion chelating assay

B. Quantitative antioxidant assays

- Reduced glutathione (GSH)
- Glutathione transferase (GST)
- Glutathione peroxidase (GPx)
- Glutathione reductase (GR)

- Superoxide dismutase (SOD)
- Catalase (CAT)
- Malondialdehyde (MDA)

A. Qualitative antioxidant assays

- ### DPPH (1,1-Diphenyl-2-picryl-hydrazyl) radical scavenging assay

  Principle:

  DPPH (1,1-Diphenyl-2-picryl-hydrazyl) is a stable free radical with purple colour. It reacts with an antioxidant compound that can donate hydrogen, and gets reduced. On scavenging, these free radicals are converted into diphenyl picryl hydrazine which is yellow in colour. This is the common principle based on which the DPPH assay is carried out (Contreras-Guzman and Strong, 1982).

  Procedure:

  In the DPPH radical scavenging assay, prepare stock solution of the drug along with various dilutions in methanol. Mix diluted solutions with methanolic solution of DPPH (0.1 mM) in 1:1 proportion and vortex the mixture. Measure the radical scavenging activity of DPPH spectro-photometrically at 517 nm after 30 min incubation in darkness at 25°C and express as the content (μg/ml) causing 50% inhibition (IC_{50}) (Blois 1958).

  Calculate the percent inhibition from the following formula.

  $$\text{Percent inhibition} = \frac{\text{Absorbance (Control)} - \text{Absorbance (Test)}}{\text{Absorbance (Control)}} \times 100$$

- ### ABTS (2,2'-azino-bis3-ethylbenzthiazoline-6-sulfonic) radical scavenging assay

  Principle:

  The colorless ABTS molecule is converted into the blue-green colored radical, ABTS•+, by oxidation of one electron. Addition of antioxidants to the preformed radical cation reduces it to ABTS, to an extent and on a time-scale depending on the antioxidant activity, the concentration of the antioxidant &

the duration of the reaction. Decrease of the absorption after addition of antioxidants is directly proportional to the number of ABTS•+ radicals (Tirzitis and Bartosz, 2010).

Procedure:

The ABTS method has been developed by Rice-Evans and Miller (1994). The procedure is as follows, prepare 7 mM ABTS solution and 2.45 mM potassium persulphate solution in distilled water respectively. Mix equal volumes of both stocks and keep at room temperature in dark for 12 to 16 hours. Dilute 700 μl of ABTS radical with 6 ml of methanol to obtain an absorbance of 0.7 ± 0.02 at 734 nm. Prepare stock solution of drug and its various dilutions in methanol. Add 10 μl of dilution sample to 1.99 ml of the blue-green ABTS radical solution. Shake the mixture vigorously and incubate in darkness for 30 minutes. The control should consist of 10 μl of methanol and 1.99 ml of ABTS radical solution. Measure the decrease in absorbance at 734 nm.

Percent inhibition was calculated from the following formula

$$\text{Percent inhibition} = \frac{\text{Absorbance (Control)} - \text{Absorbance (Test)}}{\text{Absorbance (Control)}} \times 100$$

• **Nitric oxide scavenging assay**

Principle:

Nitric oxide generated from sodium nitroprusside is measured by the Griess reduction. Sodium nitroprusside in aqueous solution at physiological pH spontaneously generates nitric oxide, which interacts with oxygen to produce nitrite ions. The nitrite ions diazotize with sulphanilic acid and couple with naphthylethylenediamine forming a complex which is pink colour measured at 546 nm. Scavengers of nitric oxide compete with the oxygen, leading to reduced production of nitric oxide (Ganapaty et al. 2007).

Procedure:

Mix 1 ml of sodium nitroprusside (10 mM) in phosphate buffer saline (PBS) (pH 7.4) with 1 ml of test samples at various concentrations dissolved in methanol and control without test sample but with equivalent amount of methanol. Incubate mixture at 25°C for 30 minutes. After 30 minutes, withdraw

1 ml of the incubated solution and mix with 1 ml of Griess reagent (1% sulphanilamide, 2% phosphoric acid and 0.1% naphthyl ethylenediamine dihydrochloride). Measure the absorbance of the pink chromophore formed during the diazotization of the nitrite with sulphanilamide and the subsequent coupling with naphthyl ethylenediamine dihydro-chloride at 546 nm (Garrat, 1964).

- ## Hydroxyl radical scavenging assay

Principle:

In this assay the scavenging activity for hydroxyl radicals is determined using Fenton reaction (Selvakumar et al. 2011).

Procedure:

Mix together 60 μl of 1.0 mM $FeCl_2$, 90 μl of 1mM 1,10-phenanthroline, 2.4 ml of 0.2 M phosphate buffer (pH 7.8), 150 μl of 0.17 M H_2O_2 and 1.5 ml of test solution with various concentrations. Add H_2O_2 to the reaction mixture in order to initiate the reaction and keep the mixture for incubation at room temperature for 5 min. After incubation read the absorbance of mixture at 560 nm using a spectrophotometer and calculate the hydroxyl radicals scavenging activity (Elizabeth and Rao, 1990).

- ## Superoxide radical scavenging activity assay

Principle:

The superoxide radicals are generated in a (phenazine methosulphate) PMS-NADH system and assayed by the reduction of nitro blue tetrazolium (NBT).

Procedure:

As per the method described by Liu, Ooi and Chang (1997), generate superoxide radicals in 1 ml of Tris HCl buffer (0.02 M, pH 8.3) containing 0.1 mM NADH, 0.1 mM NBT, 10 μM PMS and test sample. Detect the colour reaction of superoxide radicals and NBT at 560 nm using UV-Vis spectro-photometer.

- ## Hydrogen peroxide scavenging activity assay

Add test samples and standard (ascorbic acid) to 0.6 ml solution of 40 mM hydrogen peroxide (H_2O_2) in phosphate buffer pH 7.4. After 10 minutes record absorbance of H_2O_2 at 230 nm against blank solution (without H_2O_2). Calculate percent inhibition in H_2O_2 by the following expression: Percent of inhibition: $[(A_0-A_1)/A_0] \times 100$, where A_0 is the absorbance of the control and A_1 is the absorbance of the sample (Ruch at al. 1989).

• **Oxygen radical absorbance capacity (ORAC) assay**

ORAC assay is assumed to be more relevant because it utilizes a biologically relevant radical source.

Procedure:

According to the procedure reported by Cao et al. **1993**, the ORAC procedure requires an automated plate reader with 96 well plates. Conduct the analysis in phosphate buffer pH 7.4 at 37°C. Generate peroxy radical using 2,2'-azobis(2-amidino-propane) dihydrochloride which is to be prepared fresh for each run. Fluorescien is used as the substrate. Fluorescence conditions are as follows: excitation at 485 nm and emission at 520 nm. Linearity of standard curve should be between 0 to 50 μM Trolox. Express results as μM TE/g fresh mass.

• **β-Carotene/Linoleic acid (LA) assay**

Preparation:

Dissolve 0.5 mg of β-carotene in 1 ml of chloroform and add 25 μl of linoleic acid (LA) and 200 mg of Tween 20. Evaporate the chloroform under vacuum and add the residue with 100 ml of distilled water.

Procedure:

Take 500 μl of testing sample in a test tube and add 5 ml of the stock solution. Butylated hydroxytoluene (BHT) (90 μg/ml) is employed as a positive control agent. Note the absorbance of the mixture at 470 nm. Incubate the reaction mixture for 2 h at 50°C. After incubation measure the absorbance again at 470 nm (t = 120 min). Calculate the antioxidant activity as percentage inhibition of oxidation using the following equation:

% inhibition = $[1 - (\text{Absorbance sample}_0 - \text{Absorbance sample}_{120})/(\text{Absorbance control}_0 - \text{Absorbance control}_{120})] \times 100$ (Kikuzaki and Nakatani, 1993).

• **Reducing power assay**

It is another form of reducing assay which is simple and effective in analyzing the antioxidants (Selvakumar, K. et al. 2011).

Procedure:

Mix 25 μl of test sample (250 μg/ml) with 50 μl of 50 μM phosphate buffer (pH 6.6), 50 μl of 0.1% (w/v) potassium ferricyanide and incubate in a water bath at 50°C for 20 min. Add 100 μl of 1% (w/v) trichloroacetic acid solution to the mixture and centrifuge at 3000 rpm for 10 min. Remove 175 μl of the upper layer carefully and combine with 25 μl of 5 mM ferric chloride and then measure the absorbance of the reaction mixture at 700 nm. Use ascorbic acid diluted in methanol as a standard material. Express the reducing power as μg of ascorbate equivalent per mg dry weight of the test sample (Oyaizu, 1986).

- ### Ferric reducing antioxidant power (FRAP) assay

  Principle:

  The FRAP assay is simple, inexpensive, robust and fast assay which uses antioxidants as reductants in a redox linked colorimetric method to test the total antioxidant power directly (Selvakumar et al. 2011).

  Procedure:

  Mix FRAP working solution consisting of 0.3 M acetate buffer (pH=3.6), 0.01 M TPTZ (2,4,6-tripyridyl-s-triazine) in 0.04 M HCl and 0.02 M $FeCl_3 * 6H_2O$ in 10:1:1 (v/v/v), keep away from light and prepare freshly each time. Add 0.075 ml of phenols (final concentration 0.0001-0.01 mg/ml) or $FeSO_4 * 7H_2O$ (final concentration 0-1.8 μmol Fe^{2+}/ml) solution to 2.25 ml FRAP working solution and 0.225 ml of deionized water. Vortex the mixture and incubate at 37°C for 30 min in darkness. Measure absorbance at 593 nm using the spectrophotometer. Use FRAP working solution with deionized water instead of a sample as a blank (Biskup et al. 2013).

- ### Phosphomolybdenum assay

  Principle:

  This method is based on the reduction of Mo (VI) to Mo (V) by the test sample and subsequent formation of a green phosphate-Mo (V) complex in acidic condition.

  Procedure:

  Take 0.3 ml of test sample and combine with 0.3 ml of reagent solution (0.6 M sulfuric acid, 28 mM sodium phosphate and 4 mM ammonium molybdate).

Incubate the reaction mixture at 95°C for 90 minutes. Measure the absorbance of the solution at 695 nm using UV-visible spectrophotometer against blank (deionized water) after cooling to room temperature. Express the antioxidant activity as the number of gram equivalents of ascorbic acid (Kanner et al. 1994).

- **Bovine serum albumin oxidative damage assay**
  This method is used to evaluate the tendency of the antioxidants to inhibit protein oxidation.

Procedure:

Oxidize bovine serum albumin (BSA) in phosphate buffer with pH 7.4. Take 50 μl of BSA (20.0 mg/ml), 50 μl of $FeCl_2$/citric acid (4.0/4.0 mM), 50 μl of H_2O_2 (4.0 mM) and 50 μl of a sample (concentration range 62.5 to 250 μg/ml) in a 1.5 ml reaction tube and incubate in water bath at 37°C for 60 min. Butylated hydroxytoluene (BHT) is used as a positive control agent for comparison. Determine the carbonyl content of oxidised BSA in following steps; Add 0.5 ml of 2, 4-dinitrophenylhydrazine (2,4-DNPH) (10 mM in 2 N HCl) into the samples and allow to react for 60 min at room temperature, with vortexing every 15 min. Precipitate the protein by adding 0.5 ml of trichloroacetic acid (TCA) (20%) to reaction samples and followed by centrifugation for 5 min. Discard the supernatant and wash the precipitate three times with 1 ml of EtOH/EtOAc (1:1). Each wash must be followed by centrifugation and discarding of the supernatant. Dissolve the washed precipitate in 0.6 ml of guanidine (6 M in phosphate buffer, adjusted to pH 2.3 with trifluoroacetic acid (TFA), incubate at 37°C for 15 to 20 min, centrifuge and then read the absorbance at 390 nm. Results are expressed as % inhibition in carbonyl formation, relative to control (Selvakumar et al. 2011).

- **Lipid peroxidation assay**
  This is a standard method which can be performed with the help of goat liver homogenate. Add 2.8 ml of 10% goat liver homogenate, 0.1 ml of 50 mM ferrous sulphate and 0.1 ml of test sample and incubate the reaction mixture at 37°C for 30 min. Thereafter arrest the reaction by trichloroacetic acid-thiobarbituric acid (TCA-TBA) solution which comprises of 2 ml of 10% TCA-0.67% TBA made in 50% acetic acid. Add this solution to 1 ml of the reaction mixture and boil for 1 hour at 100°C. After boiling, centrifuge the mixture for 5 min at

10,000 rpm. Observe the supernatant for absorbance at 535 nm against blank. Induced vitamin E can be used as a standard. The control should consist of reaction mixture without test sample and $FeSO_4$. Lipid peroxidation percentage is calculated using the following formula, (Gow-Chin Yen et al. 1998).

$$\% \text{ ALP} = \frac{\text{Absorbance of } Fe_{2+} \text{ induced peroxidation - Absorbance of sample}}{\text{Absorbance of } Fe_{2+} \text{ induced peroxidation - Absorbance of control}} \times 100$$

- **Metal ion chelation assay**
  ▸ **Cupric ions chelation assay**

  Dilute test sample 10 times with hexamine–HCl buffer containing 10 mM KCl at pH 5.0. Mix 1 ml of prepared test sample with 1 ml of 400 μM of $CuSO_4$ prepared using hexamine–HCl buffer. Add 100 μl of 2 mM tetramethylmurexide ammonium salt (TMM) solution to this mixture subsequently and record the absorbance of the final reaction mixture at 460 and 530 nm and calculate the ratio of the absorbance at 460 and 530 nm. Determine free cupric ion concentration using a standard curve of absorbance ratio against concentration of free cupric ion. Subtract the value of free cupric ion concentration from the total amount of cupric ions to get the total concentration of chelated cupric ions and then convert to percentage (Selvakumar et al. 2011).

  ▸ **Ferrous ion chelating assay**

  Principle:

  The ferrous chelating ability of the test sample is monitored by measuring the formation of the ferrous ion-ferrozine complex.

  Procedure:

  Initiate the reaction by mixing 1.0 ml of test sample with 3.7 ml of methanol, 0.1 ml of 2 mM ferrous chloride and 0.2 ml of 5 mM ferrozine. Shake the mixture vigorously and leave to stand at room temperature for 10 minutes. Measure the absorbance of the solution at 562 nm. Calculate the percentage chelating effect on ferrozine-Fe^{2+} complex. Compare the IC_{50} values with ascorbic acid which is used as the standard (Huang and Kuo, 2000).

B. Quantitative antioxidant assays

Generally, in the quantitative antioxidant assays, the levels of reduced glutathione (GSH), and activities of enzymes such as glutathione transferase (GST), glutathione peroxidase (GPx), glutathione reductase (GR) superoxide dismutase (SOD), catalase (CAT) and lipid peroxidation are determined in various tissues of the animals such as kidney, liver, brain etc.

• ### Reduced glutathione (GSH)

Principle:

This assay is based on the reduction of glutathione (GSSG) by NADPH in the presence of glutathione reductase. In addition, 5,5'-dithiobis(2-nitrobenzoic acid) [DTNB] reacts with the reduced glutathione (GSH) formed. The reduced glutathione can then spontaneously react with DTNB to form 5-thio (2-nitrobenzoic acid) (TNB) which is measured by the increase in absorbance at 412 nm.

$$NADPH + H^+ + GSSG \xrightarrow{\quad GR \quad} NADP + 2\,GSH$$
$$GSH + DTNB \xrightarrow{\hspace{3cm}} GS\text{-}TNB + TNB$$

Procedure:

Incubate 10 μl of tissue homogenate with 200 μl of DTNB in 96 well plates for 15 min at room temperature and measure the absorbance at 412 nm using micro plate reader. Calculate the amount of GSH in the sample in microgram per ml from a standard curve obtained and represent as GSH per 100 g total tissue protein (Nishi et al. 2013).

• ### Glutathione S Transferase (GST)

Principle:

Enzyme reaction: Glutathione-SH + CDNB $\longrightarrow$ Glutathione-S-CDNB
The reaction is measured by observing the conjugation of 1-chloro, 2,4-dinitrobenzene (CDNB) with reduced glutathione (GSH). This is done by watching an increase in absorbance at 340 nm. One unit of enzyme will conjugate 10.0 nmol of CDNB with reduced glutathione per minute at 25°C.

Procedure:

Prepare stock solution of GSH in ethanol. Dissolve 100 mM CDNB in ethanol. Use PBS adjusted to pH 6.5 as the assay buffer. Prepare 1 ml of assay solution for each assay (980 μl PBS pH 6.5; 10 μl of 100 mM CDNB; 10 μl of 100 mM Glutatione). Mix the solution. For each sample and blank, place 900 μl of enzyme solution into 1.5 ml cuvette. Incubate at 30°C in spectrophotometer for 5 min. Add 100 μl PBS to the blank cuvette. Add 100 μl of sample to the cuvette and mix. Measure absorbance at 340 nm for five min (Mannervik, 1985; Boyland, 1969).

• Glutathione peroxidase (GPx)

Principle:

$$2\,GSH + H_2O_2 \xrightarrow{\text{Glutathione Peroxidase}} > GSSG + 2\,H_2O$$

$$GSSG + \beta\text{-NADPH} \xrightarrow{\text{Glutathione Reductase}} > \beta\text{-NADP} + 2\,GSH$$

GSH = Glutathione, Reduced Form GSSG = Glutathione, Oxidized Form β-NADPH = β-Nicotinamide Adenine Dinucleotide Phosphate, Reduced Form β-NADP = β-Nicotinamide Adenine Dinucleotide Phosphate, Oxidized Form

Procedure:

Prepare reaction solution by mixing 1.0 mM sodium azide solution, glutathione reductase enzyme solution, 200 mM glutathione, reduced. Mix by inversion and adjust pH to 7.0. Add reaction solution along with 10.0 mM sodium phosphate buffer in blank cuvette. Add reaction solution and glutathione peroxidase enzyme solution in test cuvette. Mix by inversion and monitor the absorbance at 340 nm. Add 0.042% (w/w) hydrogen peroxide. Immediately mix by inversion and record decrease in absorbance for approximately 5 minutes (Wendel, 1980).

• Glutathione reductase

Principle:

$$\beta\text{-NADPH} + GSSG \xrightarrow{\text{Glutathione Reductase}} > \beta\text{-NADP} + 2\,GSH$$

β-NADPH = β-Nicotinamide Adenine Dinucleotide Phosphate, Reduced Form, β-NADP = β-Nicotinamide Adenine Dinucleotide Phosphate, Oxidized Form, GSSG = Glutathione, Oxidized Form, GSH = Glutathione, Reduced Form

Procedure:

Prepare 1 ml reaction mixture consisting of 0.1 M potassium phosphate (pH 7.6), 0.1 mM NADPH, 0.5 mM EDTA, 1 mM GSSG, and 100 to 200 μl of cytosol or microsomal suspension (6 mg protein/ml). Incubate the reaction mixture at 30°C for 5 minutes before initiating the reaction by the addition of cytosol or microsomes. Determine the enzyme activity by measuring the disappearance of NADPH at 340 nm and express as nmol NADPH oxidized per minute per mg of protein (Mohandas et al. 1984).

- **Superoxide dismutase (SOD)**

Principle:

Superoxide dismutases are a class of metalloenzymes that are present in all oxygen-consuming living cells and protect organisms by controlling the concentration of superoxide ion (O_2^-) in the cell.

$$2\,O_2^- + 2H^+ \longrightarrow H_2O_2 + O_2$$

Auto-oxidation of pyrogallol in alkaline medium is inhibited by the superoxide dismutase enzyme present in the tissue homogenate, measured at 325 nm for 5 mins.

Procedure:

According to the assay described by Nishi et al. (2013), add 180 μl of phosphate buffer (pH 7.4), 10 μl of pyrogallol (2.6 mM in 10 mM HCl) and 10 μl of tissue homogenate in 96 well plates. Measure SOD activity at 325 nm for 5 mins using Elisa plate reader and express as Units per 100 g protein. One Unit of enzyme represents the enzyme activity that inhibits auto-oxidation of pyrogallol by 50%.

- **Catalase (CAT)**

Principle:

The enzyme catalyzes the decomposition of hydrogen peroxide (H_2O_2) produced by SOD to water and oxygen. The presence of catalase in a tissue sample can be determined by adding it to hydrogen peroxide and measuring the absorbance at 240 nm for 3 min. The reaction of catalase in the decomposition of H_2O_2 is as follows:

$$2\,H_2O_2 \xrightarrow{\text{Catalase}} 2H_2O + O_2$$

Procedure:

As per the procedure described by Nishi et al, (2013) assay mixture should consist of 2.9 ml hydrogen peroxide (0.019 M) and 0.1 ml tissue homogenate in a total volume of 3 ml. Changes in absorbance should be recorded at 240 nm using spectrophotometer. Catalase activity is expressed as nmol H_2O_2 consumed per min per gram of protein.

- ### Malondialdehyde (MDA)

Principle:

The method uses the reaction of malondialdehyde (MDA) and thiobarbituric acid (TBA) in the glacial acetic acid medium. MDA is considered as the major marker in lipid peroxidation. TBA is reacted with MDA which is resulting in a pink colour compound which can be determined spectrophotometrically. TBARS is now considered as a standard marker for lipid peroxidation included oxidative stress (Zeb and Ullah, 2016).

Procedure

Formation of Thiobarbituric acid reactive substances (TBARS) as a product of Lipid peroxidation is estimated in target tissues. Treat 0.2 ml of 10% tissue homogenate (0.1M phosphate buffer, pH 7.4) with 0.2 ml of sodium dodecyl sulfate (SDS), 1.5 ml acetic acid (20%, pH 3.5) and 1.5 ml of 0.8% TBA. Make the above reaction mixture up to 4 ml with distilled water, place in boiling water bath for 60 minutes and cool under tap water. Add 4 ml of butanol: pyridine (15:1 v/v) to above mixture, mix vigorously and centrifuge at room temperature for 10 minutes. Collect 200 μl of clear supernatant and measure against reference blank at 532 nm in a microplate reader. Calculate the TBARS content and express as nmol malondialde-hyde (MDA) formed per 100 gram protein (Halliwell et al., 1993; Nishi et al. 2013).

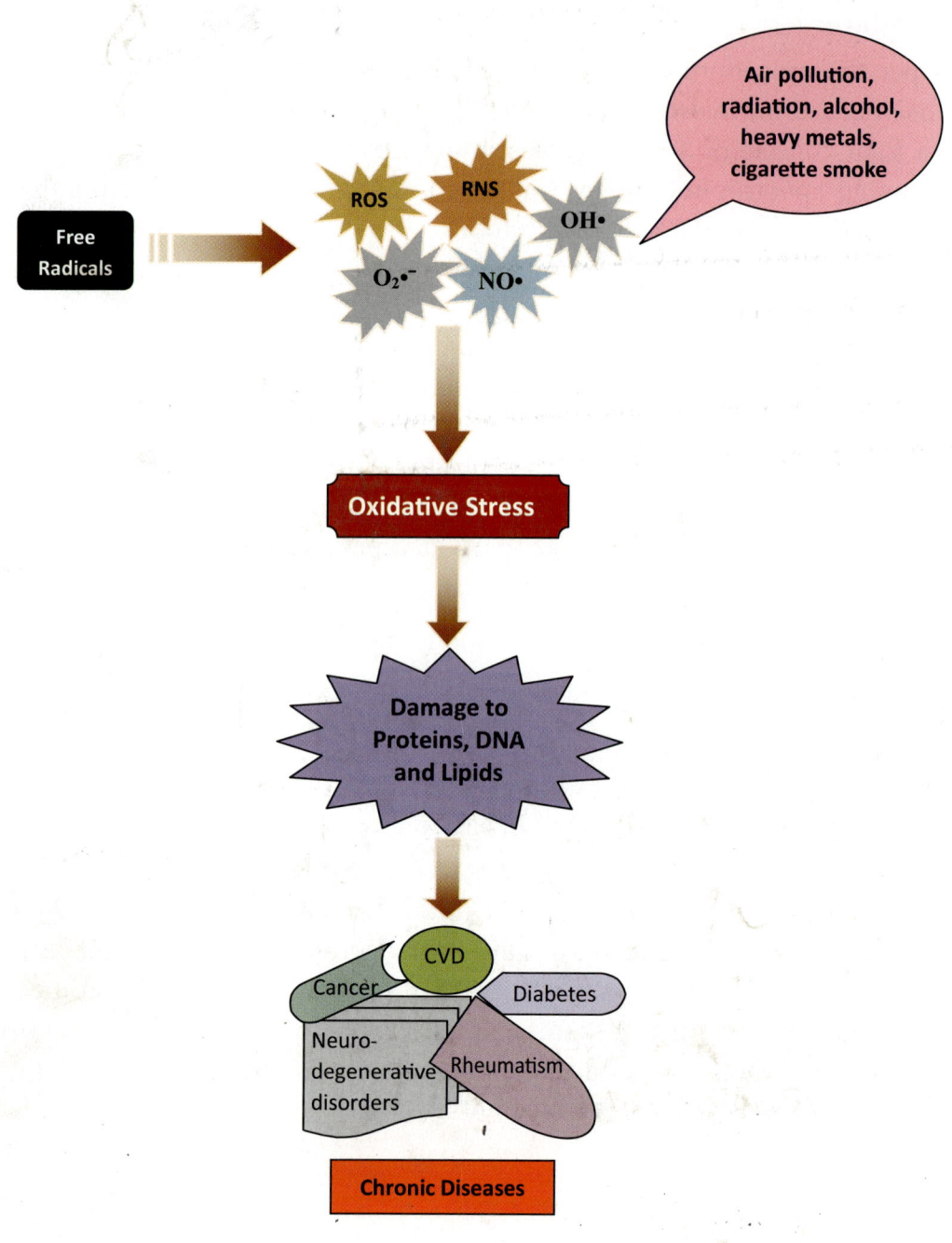

Abbreviations:

ROS: reactive oxygen species   **OH•:** hydroxyl radical   **NO•:** nitric oxide radical
RNS: reactive nitrogen species $O_2•^-$: superoxide radical   **CVD:** cardiovascular disorders

Fig 10.1: Role of oxidative stress and antioxidants in the genesis of diseases (Mazumdar et al. 2012)

References:

1. Mazumdar, P.M.; Rathinavelusamy, P.; Sasmal, D. Role of antioxidants in phytomedicine with special reference to anti-diabetic herbs. Asian Pacific Journal of Tropical Disease. **2012**, 2(2), S969-S979.

2. Surveswaran, S.; Cai, Y.; Corke, H.; Sun, H. Systematic evaluation of natural phenolic antioxidants from 133 Indian medicinal plants. Food Chemistry. **2007**, 102, 938-953.

3. Selvakumar, K.; Madhan, R.; Srinivasan, G.; Baskar, V. Antioxidant assays in pharmacological research. Asian Journal of Pharmaceutical Technology. **2011**, 1(4), 99-103.

4. Auddy, B.; Ferreira, M.; Blasina, F.; Lafon, L.; Arredondo, F.; Dajas, F.; Tripathi, P.C.; Seal, T.; Mukherjee, B. Screening of antioxidant activity of three Indian medicinal plants, traditionally used for the management of neurodegenerative diseases. Journal of Ethnopharmacology. **2003**, 84 (2-3), 131-8.

5. Contreras-Guzman, E.S. and Strong, F.C. Determination of tocopherols (Vitamin E) by reduction of cupric ion. JAOAC. **1982**, 65:1215-1222.

6. Blois, M.S. Antioxidant determinations by the use of a stable free radical. Nature. **1958**, 181:1199-1200.

7. Rice-Evans, C.; Miller, N.J. Total antioxidant status in plasma and body fluids. Methods Enzymol. **1994**, 234:279-293.

8. Ganapaty, S.; Chandrashekhar, V.M.; Chitme, H.R.; Lakashami Narsu, M. Free radical scavenging activity of gossypin and nevadensin: an in-vitro evaluation. Indian Journal of Pharmacology. **2007**, 39(6), 281-283.

9. Garrat, D.C. The quantitative analysis of drugs. Vol. 3. Chapman and Hall ltd; Japan; 456-458.

10. Elizabeth, K. and Rao, M.N.A. Oxygen radical scavenging activity of curcumin. Int J Pharmaceut. **1990**, 58:237-240.

11. Liu, F.; Ooi, V. E. C.; Chang, T. Free radical scavenging activity of mushroom polysaccharide extract. Life Science. **1997**, 60, 731–763.

12. Ruch, R.J.; Cheng, S.J.; Klaunig, J.E. Prevention of cytotoxicity and inhibition of intercellular communication by antioxidant catechins isolated from Chinese green tea. Carcinogenesis. **1989**; 10:1003-1008.

13. Cao, G.; Alessino, H.M.; Cutler, R.G. Oxygen radical absorbance capacity assay for antioxidants. Free Radical Biology and Medicine. **1993**, 14(3):303-311.

14. Oyaizu, M. Studies on products of browning reaction: antioxidative activity of products of browning reaction prepared from glucosamine. Jpn J Nutr. **1986**, 44:307-315.

15. Biskup, I.; Golonka, I.; Gamian, A.; Sroka, Z. Antioxidant activity of selected phenols estimated by ABTS and FRAP methods. Postepy Hig med Dosw. **2013**, 67, 958-963.

16. Kaneer, J. et al. Natural antioxidants in grapes and wines. J Agri Food Chem. **1994**, 42: 64-69.

17. Huang, S. and Kuo, J.C. Concentrations and antioxidant activity of Anserine and Carnosine in poultry meat extracts treated with demineralization and papain. Proc Natl Sci Counc Repub China B. **2000**, 24(4), 193-201.

18. Kikuzaki H, Nakatani N. Antioxidant effects of some ginger constituents. J Food Sci. **1993**; 58:1407–1410.

19. Gow-Chin Yen and Chiu-Luan Hseih. Antioxidant activity of extracts from Du-zhong (Eucommia ulmoides) toward various lipid peroxidation models in vitro. J Agri Food Chem. **1998**, 46: 3952-3957.

20. Mohandas, J.; Marshall, J.J.; Duggin, G.G.; Horvath, J.S. Tiller, D.G. Low activities of glutathione-related enzymes as factors in the genesis of urinary bladder cancer. Cancer Res. **1984**, 44: 5086-5091.

21. Nishi; Ahad, A.; Kumar, P. Protective effect of chlorogenic acid against diabetic nephropathy in high fat diet/streptozotocin induced type-2 diabetic rats. Int J Pharm Pharm Sci. **2013**, 5,489-495.

22. Mannervik, B. The isozymes of Glutatione Transferase. Adv. Enzymol. Relat. Areas Mol. Biol. **1985**, 57, 357-417.

23. Boyland, E. and Chasseaud, L.F. The Role of Glutathione and Glutathione S Transferase in Mercaptic Acid Biosynthesis. Adv. Enzymol. **1969**, 32 173 – 219.

24. Wendel, A. Enzymatic Basis of Detoxication, **1980**, Volume 1, p. 333, Academic Press, NY

25. Zeb, A. and Ullah, F. A simple spectrophotometric method for the determination of thiobarbituric acid reactive substances in fried fast foods. Journal of Analytical Methods in Chemistry. **2016**, **2016**, 1-5. http://dx.doi.org/10.1155/2016/9412767

26. Halliwell, B. and Chirico, S. Lipid peroxidation: its mechanism, measurement, and significance. Am J Clin Nutr. **1993**, 57:715S-724S.

11 TOXICOLOGICAL METHODS AND TECHNIQUES

IMPORTANCE OF TOXICOLOGY

Toxicity testing plays a critical role prior to the evaluation and development of drugs for human use. Toxicity testing helps to determine the deleterious and toxic reactions that the test substance is likely to produce in animal studies. The prime objective of toxicity studies is to determine its safety as well as the toxic manifestations that the test substance can produce.

Attention to the desperate need to toxicity study, came into existence in early 1960s, when Thalidomide proved to be a teratogenic substance, thereby leading children born with several birth defects. It was after this tragic incident, that there was a worldwide agreement to perform toxicity testing, to prevent any further adverse toxic effects.

The importance of toxicity broadly include in the following factors:
- To obtain a dose response curve
- To ensure the safety of new chemicals such as pesticides, food additives or drugs, before they are marketed.
- To investigate the mechanism(s) of the toxic effect.
- To develop or validate any new method of toxicity testing specially *in-vitro* condition, rather than *in-vivo*.
- To correlate the possible hazards on human, by exposure of animals to high dose of drugs.

Toxicity testing can be classified as follows:

1) Acute toxicity testing by different routes :
   a) Oral
   b) Inhalation
   c) Dermal

2) Subchronic toxicity testing
3) Chronic toxicity testing
4) Mutagenicity testing
5) Carcinogenecity testing
6) Reproduction toxicity testing
7) Toxicokinetics
8) Neurotoxicity studies
9) Embryotoxicity studies

Brief explanations of each of these testing methods are as follows:

1) Acute toxicity testing:

This testing involves the evaluation of single dose hazards. It is basically used to obtain the LD_{50} value of a test substance. LD_{50} is a dose that kills 50% of the animals. LD_{50} is an essential parameter of toxicity studies.

Importance of acute toxicity testing are:
- To find out the target organ toxicity
- To establish safety guidelines for the development as well as for the toxicity of chemicals.
- To serve as an index for dose selection for long term toxicity studies.
- To serve as basis to perform other screening models.
- To help classify the toxicity grade/category of the chemical and to assign the proper labeling of the chemical entity.

In general, acute toxicity testing is carried out using two different animal species. The drug is administered at various dose levels and observed for duration of 14 days. After the observation period the animals are sacrificed and histopathological studies are performed.

The methods used are namely:

i) The fixed dose procedure (FDP)(OECD guideline 420): In FDP, the drug is administered at fixed dose levels of 5,50,500 and 2000 mg/kg.

ii) Acute toxic class method (ATC)(OECD guideline 423): In ATC, the method uses a sequential increase in dose, using 3 animals of same sex (preferably female) in each step.

iii) Up down procedure (UDP)(OECD guideline 425): This method involves single dose administration in animals in a sequential manner at an interval of 48 hours.

A) Acute toxicity testing for inhalation: This is done for aerosol like formulations. The animals are exposed to the preparation for a total period of 4 hours and observed for a period of 14 days.

B) Acute toxicity testing of topical preparations: Topical preparations are subjected to eye irritation and skin irritation testing. The Draize test is performed to evaluate the hazards using rabbits and guinea pigs.

In Draize eye irritation test, 0.5 ml of the ophthalmic preparation is instilled into the conjunctiva of eye of the animal, and then the animal is restrained for 4 hours. The animal is then observed for a period of 14 days for any toxic manifestations (such as lacrimation, redness, edema etc).

In Draize skin irritation test, 0.5 g of the dermal preparation like creams, pastes and lotions is applied onto the animal's shaven dorsal part of unit area of the body and observed for 14 days.

2) Subchronic toxicity testing:

In this study, the test drug is administered for a period of 90 days. Both rodents and non-rodents are used to evaluate the subchronic toxicity profile of the drug.

3) Chronic toxicity testing:

This study is used to evaluate the long term toxic effect of a test substance in animals. The duration for study varies from 6 months to 1 year or more. The study requires conducting the test on a minimum of one rodent and one non-rodent species.

4) Mutagenecity testing:

This test is used to evaluate the toxic effect of a drug substance on the base sequence of DNA. The DNA changes may include insertion, deletion, inversions, duplication and translocation of DNA bases.

Carcinogenesis is a type of mutagenecity that is caused by mutation of the tumor suppressor gene. Mutagenecity test is first done *in-vitro*, using specific bacterial species (e.g. Salmonella typhi) and mammalian cells (such as mammalian cell hypoxanthine phosphoribosyl transferase (HPRT) gene). *In-vivo* mutagenecity studies are done on transgenic animals, since they are more suitable in determining the toxicity of the test substance.

5) Carcinogenecity testing:

These tests are carried out in both rodent and non-rodent animal species. The test is carried throughout a large portion of the animal's life span. During and after completion of the study, the animals are checked for development of tumors and also other signs of toxicity. The animals at the end of the study are sacrificed and pathological/architectural changes are recorded.

6) Reproduction toxicity testing:

This study is done to ascertain the effect of drug on the reproduction process.

i) **One generation reproduction toxicity testing:** Rodents are the preferred species for this study. The test substance is to be administered to both male and female animals. In males, the drug is administered for duration of one complete spermatogenic cycle and in females for two complete estrous cycles. After the completion of duration of drug administration, animals are allowed to mate. Further, the drug is administered during gestation as well as nursing. The sperm of male animals are analyzed. On parturtion, the number of dead and live pups are noted and observed for first 4 days. The animals and pups are sacrificed and subjected to histopathological evaluation.

7) Toxicokinetics:

It is a branch of pharmacokinetics that deals with the study of the kinetics of drugs at higher doses. These tests reveal the metabolism and excretion pattern of chemical substances. Toxicokinetics testing can be performed in rodents, dogs, swine and primates. These studies can be done using *in-vitro* cell lines as well.

8) Neurotoxicity studies:

This study helps in understanding the effect of test substance on the central nervous system. They characterize the neurotoxic effect by the observation of loss of cognitive functions, sensing defects and impaired learning ability as well as neuropathological changes.

The test drug is to be administered for 28 days or more than 90 days, and the neurological changes are noted. Various *in-vitro* neurotoxicity models (such as neuroblastoma cell line and chick brain retina primary monolayer and re-aggregate cultures) have been developed and are recommended.

9) Embryotoxicity studies:

Rodents (rabbits) are preferred for these testing. The administration of the substance is carried out between the 8th and 14th day of the gestation period. On 21st day of the study, a caesarean section is performed under light anesthesia and various biological and pathological parameters of the fetus are studied. Although *in-vivo* testing is preferred, in-*vitro* techniques using suitable cell lines can also be performed to study teratogenecity.

ROLE OF REGULATORY AGENCIES IN TOXICOLOGY:

The regulatory bodies play a vital role in the conductance of toxicity testing. They provide us the various guidelines to successfully carry out the investigation and also prevent any un-ethical testing from being conducted. They require the toxicity testing to be carried out in minimum three doses (low, intermediate and high dose) estimated on the basis of LD_{50} in the animals and the effect of toxicity compared with the control group.

The regulatory bodies are:
*   International Conference on Harmonization (ICH)
*   World Health Organization (WHO)
*   Organization for Economic Co-operation and development (OECD)
*   Food and Drug administration (FDA)

The Organization for Economic Co-operation and Development (OECD) Guidelines are a unique tool for assessing the potential effects of chemicals on human health and the environment. Accepted internationally as standard methods for safety testing, the guidelines are used by professionals in industry, academia and government involved in the testing and assessment of chemicals (industrial chemicals, pesticides, personal care products, etc.). These guidelines are regularly updated with the assistance of thousands of national experts from OECD member countries.

Important definitions:

1. **Acute oral toxicity** refers to those adverse effects occurring following oral administration of a single dose of a substance, or multiple doses given within 24 hours.

2. **Dose** is the amount of test substance administered. Dose is expressed as weight of test substance per unit weight of test animal (e.g. mg/kg).

3. **Dosage** is a general term comprising of dose, its frequency and the duration of dosing.

4. **LD$_{50}$** (median lethal oral dose) is a statistically derived single dose of a substance that can be expected to cause death in 50 per cent of animals when administered by the oral route. The LD$_{50}$ value is expressed in terms of weight of test substance per unit weight of test animal (mg/kg).

5. **NOAEL** is the abbreviation for no-observed-adverse-effect level. This is the highest dose level where no adverse treatment-related findings are observed due to treatment.

6. **LOAEL** is the abbreviation for lowest observed adverse effect level.

7. **Delayed death:** An animal does not die or appear moribund within 48 hours but dies later during the 14-day observation period.

8. **Impending death:** It is described as a stage when moribund state or death is expected prior to the next planned time of observation. Some of the signs indicative of this state are convulsions, lateral position, recumbence and tremor.

9. **Moribund status:** It is defined as being in a state of dying or inability to survive, even if treated.

10. **Satellite group:** A group of animals used in the toxicity study to monitor the reversibility of any toxicological changes induced by the chemical under investigation. Usually satellite groups are used for the highest dose level of the study and control.

ICH SAFETY GUIDELINES

S1A-S1C-Carcinogenicity studies
S2-Genotoxicity studies
S3A-S3B-Toxicokinetics and Pharmacokinetics
S4-Toxicity testing
S5-Reproductive toxicology
S6-Biotechnological products
S7A-S7B-Pharmacology studies
S8-Immunotoxicology studies
S9-Nonclinical evaluation for anticancer pharmaceuticals
S10-Photosafety evaluation
S11-Nonclinical safety testing

Box 1: OECD GUIDELINES FOR THE TESTING OF CHEMICALS

1. General toxicity guidelines:

Test No. 420: Acute Oral Toxicity: Fixed Dose Procedure

Test No. 425: Acute Oral Toxicity: Up-and-Down Procedure

Test No. 423: Acute Oral toxicity: Acute Toxic Class Method

Test No. 407: Repeated Dose 28-day Oral Toxicity Study in Rodents

Test No. 408: Repeated Dose 90-Day Oral Toxicity Study in Rodents

Test No. 409: Repeated Dose 90-Day Oral Toxicity Study in Non-Rodents

Test No. 452: Chronic Toxicity Studies

Test No. 453: Combined Chronic Toxicity/Carcinogenicity Studies

2. Dermal toxicity:

Test No. 402: Acute Dermal Toxicity

Test No. 404: Acute Dermal Irritation/Corrosion

Test No. 410: Repeated Dose Dermal Toxicity: 21/28-day Study

Test No. 411: Subchronic Dermal Toxicity: 90-day Study

Test No. 442E: *In-vitro* Skin Sensitization Human Cell Line Activation Test (H-CLAT)

Test No. 431: *In-vitro* skin corrosion: reconstructed human epidermis (RHE) test method

Test No. 404: Acute Dermal Irritation/Corrosion

Test No. 430: *In-vitro* Skin Corrosion: Transcutaneous Electrical Resistance Test Method (TER)

Test No. 435: *In-vitro* Membrane Barrier Test Method for Skin Corrosion

Test No. 439: *In-vitro* Skin Irritation: Reconstructed Human Epidermis Test Method

Test No. 442C: In Chemical Skin Sensitization Direct Peptide Reactivity Assay (DPRA)

Test No. 442D: *In-vitro* Skin Sensitization ARE-Nrf2 Luciferase Test Method

Test No.429: Skin Sensitization Local Lymph Node Assay

Test No. 442A: Skin Sensitization Local Lymph Node Assay: DA

Test No. 442B: Skin Sensitization Local Lymph Node Assay: BrdU-ELISA

Test No. 427: Skin Absorption: *In-vivo* Method

Test No. 428: Skin Absorption: *In-vitro* Method

Test No. 432: *In-vitro* 3T3 NRU Phototoxicity Test

3. Reproductive toxicity

Test No. 421: Reproduction/Developmental Toxicity Screening Test

Test No. 422: Combined Repeated Dose Toxicity Study with the Reproduction/ Developmental Toxicity Screening Test

Test No. 443: Extended One-Generation Reproductive Toxicity Study

Test No. 426: Developmental Neurotoxicity Study

Test No. 414: Prenatal Development Toxicity Study

Test No. 416: Two-Generation Reproduction Toxicity

Test No. 415: One-Generation Reproduction Toxicity Study

4. Mutagenicity and carcinogenicity

Test No. 471: Bacterial Reverse Mutation Test

Test No. 473: *In-vitro* Mammalian Chromosomal Aberration Test

Test No. 474: Mammalian Erythrocyte Micronucleus Test

Test No. 475: Mammalian Bone Marrow Chromosomal Aberration Test

Test No. 476: *In-vitro* Mammalian Cell Gene Mutation Tests using the HPRT and XPRT genes

Test No. 478: Rodent Dominant Lethal Test

Test No. 483: Mammalian Spermatogonial Chromosomal Aberration Test

Test No. 486: Unscheduled DNA Synthesis (UDS) Test with Mammalian Liver Cells in vivo

Test No. 487: *In-vitro* Mammalian Cell Micronucleus Test

Test No. 489: *In-vivo* Mammalian Alkaline Comet Assay

Test No. 490: *In-vitro* Mammalian Cell Gene Mutation Tests Using the Thymidine Kinase Gene

Test No. 488: Transgenic Rodent Somatic and Germ Cell Gene Mutation Assays

Test No. 451: Carcinogenicity Studies

Test No. 479: Genetic Toxicology: In vitro Sister Chromatid Exchange Assay in Mammalian Cells

Test No. 480 : Genetic Toxicology: *Saccharomyces cerevisiae*, Gene Mutation Assay

Test No. 481: Genetic Toxicology: *Saccharomyces cerevisiae*, Mitotic Recombination Assay

Test No. 482: Genetic Toxicology: DNA Damage and Repair, Unscheduled DNA Synthesis in Mammalian Cells *in-vitro*

Test No. 484: Genetic Toxicology: Mouse Spot Test

Test No. 485: Genetic toxicology, Mouse Heritable Translocation Assay

Test No. 477: Genetic Toxicology: Sex-Linked Recessive Lethal Test in *Drosophila melanogaster*

5. Ocular toxicity

Test No. 405: Acute Eye Irritation/Corrosion

Test No. 491: Short Time Exposure *In-vitro* Test Method for Identifying

(i) Chemicals Inducing Serious Eye Damage and

(ii) Chemicals Not Requiring Classification for Eye Irritation or Serious Eye Damage

Test No. 492: Reconstructed human Cornea-like Epithelium (RhCE) test method for identifying chemicals not requiring classification and labeling for eye irritation or serious eye damage

Test No. 437: Bovine Corneal Opacity and Permeability Test Method for Identifying

(i) Chemicals Inducing Serious Eye Damage and

(ii) Chemicals Not Requiring Classification for Eye Irritation or Serious Eye Damage

Test No. 438: Isolated Chicken Eye Test Method for Identifying

(i) Chemicals Inducing Serious Eye Damage and

(ii) Chemicals Not Requiring Classification for Eye Irritation or Serious Eye Damage

Test No. 460: Fluorescein Leakage Test Method for Identifying Ocular Corrosives and Severe Irritants

6. Test No. 417: Toxicokinetics

7. Inhalational toxicity

Test No. 403: Acute Inhalation Toxicity

Test No. 412: Sub-acute Inhalation Toxicity: 28-Day Study

Test No. 413: Subchronic Inhalation Toxicity: 90-Day Study

Test No. 436: Acute Inhalation Toxicity – Acute Toxic Class Method

8. Test No. 424: Neurotoxicity Study in Rodents

Initial considerations:

The testing laboratory should consider all available information on the test substance prior to conducting the study. Such information will include the identity and chemical structure of the test substance; its physical chemical properties; the results of any other *in-vitro* or *in-vivo* toxicity tests on the substance; toxicological data on structurally related substances or similar mixtures; and the anticipated use(s) of the substance. This information is useful to determine the relevance of the test for the protection of human health and the environment, and will help in the selection of an appropriate starting dose.

General conditions for toxicity testing:

A. Selection of animal species

The preferred rodent species is the rat, although other rodent species may be used. Normally females are used. This is because literature surveys of conventional LD_{50} tests show that usually there is little difference in sensitivity between the sexes, but in those cases where differences are observed, females are generally slightly more sensitive. However, if knowledge of the toxicological or toxicokinetic properties of structurally related chemicals indicates that males are likely to be more sensitive then this sex should be used. When the test is conducted in males, adequate justification should be provided.

Healthy young adult animals of commonly used laboratory strains should be employed. Females should be nulliparous and non-pregnant. Each animal, at the commencement of its dosing, should be between 8 and 12 weeks old and its weight should fall in an interval within ± 20% of the mean weight of any previously dosed animals.

B. Animal housing and feeding conditions

The temperature of the experimental animal room should be 22°C (±3°C). Although the relative humidity should be at least 30% and preferably not exceed 70% other than during room cleaning the aim should be 50-60%.

Lighting should be artificial, the sequence being 12 hours light, 12 hours dark. For feeding, conventional laboratory diets may be used with an unlimited supply of drinking water. Animals may be group-caged by dose, but the number of animals per cage must not interfere with clear observations of each animal.

C. Preparation of doses

In general test substances should be administered in a constant volume over the range of doses to be tested by varying the concentration of the dosing preparation. In rodents, the volume should not normally exceed 1 mL/100 g of body weight: however, in the case of aqueous solutions 2 mL/100 g body weight can be considered. Doses must be prepared shortly prior to administration unless the stability of the preparation over the period during which it will be used is known and shown to be acceptable.

References:

1. Wooley A. A guide to practical toxicology, evaluation, prediction and risk, 2nd edition, Informa Health care, New York, London, 2008.

2. Cunny H., Hodgson E., Toxicity testing. In: Hodgson E(ed). A textbook on modern toxicology 3rd edition. A John Wiley and Sons. Inc publication.353-384.

3. Walum E. Acute oral toxicity. Environ Health Perpect 1998;106;497-503.

4. Stallard N, Whitehead A, Reducing animal numbers in the fixed dose procedure. Human Exp Toxicol. 1995;14:315-323.

CARDIOPROTECTIVE AND NEPHROPROTECTIVE *(in-vivo)* SCREENING METHODS

Isoproterenol - Induced Cardiotoxicity

Induction of Myocardial Ischemia:

Isoproterenol is to be dissolved in normal saline and 85 mg/kg dose of isoproterenol injected subcutaneously to rats at an interval of 24 hours for two days to induce experimental myocardial ischemia.

Post-treatment Investigation:

Twenty four hours after the last injection of isoproterenol, the animals should be euthanized under light anesthesia. Blood is to be collected from jugular vein and serum must be separated by centrifugation for 10 min at 4°C. The hearts should be dissected out, frozen with liquid nitrogen and preserved at -20°C. Before analysis, hearts must be thawed at room temperature and homogenate should be prepared in 0.1 M Tris HCl buffer (pH 7.4). The homogenate should be centrifuged for 10 min at 4°C and the supernatant must be used for enzyme estimation. A portion of heart should be preserved in 10% formalin (pH 7.2) and subjected to histopathological studies.

Evaluation Parameters

1. Organ body weight indices of hearts

2. Biochemical Parameters:
   In serum: Alanine aminotransferase (ALT), aspartate aminotransferase (AST), lactate dehydrogenase (LDH) and creatine kinase (CK) must be estimated. The serum lipid profile consisting of total cholesterol, tryglycerides, HDL, cholesterol, LDL cholesterol and VLDL cholesterol should be evaluated. Standard biochemical kits can be used for these evaluations.

In heart homogenate: Alanine aminotransferase (ALT), aspartate aminotransferase (AST), lactate dehydrogenase (LDH) and creatin kinase (CK) along with myocardial thiobarbituric acid reactive substances (TBARS) are estimated. Reduced glutathione (GSH), glutathione reductase (GR), glutathione-S-transferase (GST), glutathione peroxidase (GPOX), superoxide dismutase (SOD) and catalase (CAT) levels should be measured in heart homogenate using standardised assay procedures.

Doxorubicin - induced Cardiotoxicity and Nephrotoxicity:

Male Sprague Dawley rats weighing between 160-180 g should be used for this study.

Induction of Cardiotoxicity and Nephrotoxicity:

Freeze dried powder of Doxorubicin injection should be reconstituted with water for injection. Doxorubicin should be administered intraperitoneally to rats for induction of experimental cardiotoxicity and nephrotoxicity.

Post-treatment Investigation

Twenty four hours after the injection of Doxorubicin, the animals are euthanized under light anesthesia. Blood is to be collected from jugular vein and serum must be separated by centrifugation. The hearts and kidneys must be dissected out, frozen with liquid nitrogen and preserved at -20°C. Before analysis, hearts and kidneys must be thawed at room temperature. Heart homogenate must be prepared in 1% KCl solution. The homogenate must be centrifuged and the supernatant should be used for enzyme estimation. A portion of heart and kidneys tissue must be preserved in 10% formalin (pH 7.2) and subjected to histopathological studies.

Parameters to be evaluated

1. Organ body weight indices of hearts and kidneys
2. Biomedical Parameters

   In kidney homogenate: Renal antioxidant enzymes viz. superoxide dismutase (SOD), Catalase (CAT) and glutathione peroxide (GPOX) must be estimated. Reduced glutathione (GSH) and renal thiobarbituric acid reactive substances (TBARS) must be estimated.

BIOCHEMICAL PARAMETERS: PRINCIPLE AND METHODOLOGY

A) Marker Enzymes

1. **Quantitative determination of aspartate aminotransferase (AST) activity**

   Principle:

   AST (GOT) catalyzes the following reactions:

   $$\alpha\text{-Ketoglutarate} + \text{L-Aspartate} \xrightarrow{\text{GOT}} \text{Glutamate} + \text{Oxaloacetate}$$

   $$\text{Oxaloacetate} + \text{NADH} + \text{H}^+ \xrightarrow{\text{MDH}} \text{Malate} + \text{NAD}^+$$

   The rate of NADH consumption is measured photometrically and is directly proportional to the GOT activity.

   Procedure:

   Reagent 1 (Reagent solution) and Reagent 2 (start reagent) are mixed in 4:1 proportion to prepare the reaction solution. 500 μl of reaction solution is then mixed with 50 μl of serum and after approximately 1 minute, the decrease in absorption is measured every min (for 3 min) at 340 nm.

   Calculation:

   Enzyme activity (U/I) = (Δ A/min) × 1746

2. **Quantitative Determination of Alanine aminotransferase (ALT) activity**

   Principle:

   ALT (GPT) catalyzes the following reaction:

   $$2\text{-Oxoglutarate} + \alpha\text{-Ketoglutaric acid} \xrightarrow{\text{GPT}} \text{Glutamate} + \text{Pyruvic acid}$$

   $$\text{Pyruvic acid} + \text{NADH} + \text{H}^+ \xrightarrow{\text{LDH}} \text{Lactic acid} + \text{NAD}^+$$

   The rate of NADH consumption is measured photometrically and is directly proportional to the ALT activity.

   Procedure:

   Reagent 1 (Reagent solution) and Reagent 2 (start reagent) are mixed in 4:1 proportion to prepare the reaction solution. 500 μl of reaction solution is then mixed with 50 μl of serum and after approximately 1 minute, the decrease in absorption is measured every min (for 3 min) at 340 nm.

Calculation:
Enzyme activity (U/I) = (Δ A/min) $\times$ 1746

3. **Quantitative Determination of Lactose dehydrogenase (LDH) activity**
   Principle:
   LDH catalyzes the oxidation of lactate to pyruvate in the presence of NAD^+ which subsequently gets reduced to NADH.

$$\text{Lactic acid} + NAD^+ \overset{LDH}{\rightleftharpoons} \text{Pyruvic acid} + NADH + H^+$$

The rate of NADH formation measured at 340 nm is directly proportional to to serum LDH activity.

Procedure:
Reagent in each vial is reconstituted with 1 ml distilled water. 1 ml reagent i.e. pipetted out into test tube and pre-warmed at 37°C for 3 min. Spectrophotometer reading is set at zero with water at 340 nm. 25 μl of serum is added to the reagent, mixed and incubated at 37°C for 1 min. Absorbance is recorded after 1 min and reading is repeated every minute for the next two minutes. Average absorbance difference per minute (Δ Ab / min) is calculated.

Calculation:
Unit definition: One international unit (IU/L) is the amount of enzyme that will reduce one micromole of NAD per minute at specific temperature.
IU/L = Δ Ab/min. $\times$ 6592

4. **Quantitative Determination of Creatine kinase (CK) activity**

$$\text{Creatine phosphate} + \text{ADP} \overset{CK}{\rightleftharpoons} \text{Creatine} + \text{ATP}$$

$$\text{ATP} + \text{D- Glucose} \overset{HK}{\rightleftharpoons} \text{Glucose-6- Phosphate} + \text{ADP}$$

$$\text{Glucose-6-phosphate} + \text{NAD} \overset{G\text{-}6\text{-}PDH}{\rightleftharpoons} \text{6-Phosphogluconate} + NADH + H^+$$

The rate of NADP formation measured at 340 nm is directly proportional to serum CK activity.

Procedure:

Reagent in each vial is reconstituted with 1 ml distilled water. 1 ml reagent is pipetted out into test tube and pre-warmed at 37°C for 3 min. Spectrophotometer reading is set at zero with water at 340 nm. 25 μl of serum is added to the reagent, mixed and incubated at 37°C for 1 min. Absorbance is recorded after 1 min and reading is repeated every minute for the next two minutes. Average absorbance difference per minute (Δ Ab / min) is calculated.

Calculation

IU/L = Δ Ab/min. $\times$ 6592

B. Parameters to Evaluate Oxidative stress

1. Quantitative Determination of Superoxide Dismutase (SOD) activity:

Principle:

$$2O_2^- + 2H^+ \xrightleftharpoons{\text{SOD}} H_2O_2 + O_2$$

Procedure:

Measurement of SOD activity is carried out spectrophotometrically by the method of Marklund and Marklund (1974). The assay medium in a total volume of 1.0 ml contained: 50 mM sample, 30 mM EDTA, 100 mM potassium phosphate buffer (pH 8.2) and 0.2 mM pyrogallol. Autoxidation of pyrogallol is monitored at 420 nm for 3 min in the absence and presence sample and inhibition of pyrogallol autoxidation by sample in this case tissue homogenate, is calculated. One unit of the enzyme activity is defined as the amount which produced 50% inhibition of pyrogallol autoxidation under the standard assay conditions.

2. Quantitative determination of Catalase activity:

Principle:

$$2H_2O_2 \xrightleftharpoons{\text{Catalase}} 2H_2O + O_2$$

Procedure:

A 10 μl of supernatant is added to a quartz cuvette containing 1.990 ml of 10 mM H_2O_2 solution prepared in 50 mM phosphate buffer, pH 7.0. change in absorbance are read at 240 nm for 1 min. using the reaction time interval (Δt) of absorbance (A1 and A2). The following equation is used to calculate the rate constant (K):K = (2.3/Δt) × log (A1/A2). The specific activity of the enzyme is expressed as K/mg protein.

Calculations:

Enzyme activity K =(2.3/Δt) × log (A1/A2)

3. **Quantitative determination of Glutathione Peroxidase (GPOX) Activity: (Beutler, 1975, Maehly and Chance, 1954)**

Principle:

$$\text{Reduced Guaiacol} + H_2O_2 \underset{}{\overset{GPOX}{\rightleftharpoons}} 2H_2O + \text{Oxidized Guaiacol}$$

Procedure:

For GPOX, the oxidation of Guaiacol is measured by following the increase in absorbance at 470 nm for 1 min. The assay mixture contained 50 mM phosphate buffer (pH=7), 0.1 mM EDTA, 10 mM Guaiacol and 10 mM H_2O_2 as described by Chance and Maehly (1995). GPOX activity is expressed as μmol of tetraguaiacol formed mg protein^{-1} min^{-1}.

Calculation:

Enzyme activity (U/I)=(ΔA/min.) × factor

4. **Quantitative determination of Glutathione Reductase (GR) Activity: (Caerlberg and Mannervik,1979; Shaedle and Bassham, 1977)**

Principle:

$$GSSG + NADPH + H^+ \underset{}{\overset{GR}{\rightleftharpoons}} 2GSH + NADP^+$$

The above reaction is shown as reversible, but the reaction forming GSH is strongly favored. Activity is measured by following the decrease in absorbance due to oxidation of NADPH.

Procedure:

GR activity is measured by monitoring the decrease in absorbance at 340nm for 1 min. The reaction mixture contained 50 mM Tris-HCl buffer (pH 7.5), 0.5 mM GSSG, 0.1 mM EDTA, 3mM $MgCl_2$ and 0.15 mM NADPH as described by Shaedle and Bassham, 1977. Activity is expressed as μmol of NADPH oxidized mg protein^{-1} min^{-1} .

Calculation:

Enzyme activity (U/I)=(ΔA/min.) $\times$ factor

5. **Quantitative determination of Glutathione S-Transferase (GST) Activity: (Habig et al, 1974)**

Principle:

$$GSH + CDNB \overset{GST}{\rightleftharpoons} GS\text{-}DNB + H^+ + Cl^-$$

The GST-catalyzed formation of CDNB-GSH produces a dinitro-phenyl thioether, which can be detected at 340 nm. One unit of GST activity is defined as the amount of enzyme producing 1 mmol of CDNB-GSH conjugate/min.

Procedure:

GST activity is measured by following the changes in the absorbance of 340 nm for 1 min in a mixture containing 100 mM sodium phosphate buffer (pH 6.5), 1 mM GSH and 1 mM CDNB. The activity of GST is expressed as μmol of dinitro-phenyl glutathione formed mg protein^{-1} min^{-1} .

6. **Quantitative determination of Reduced Glutathione (GSH) (Ellman, 1959)**

Principle:

$$GSH + DTNB \rightleftharpoons GSSG + TNB$$

The catalytic amounts Glutathione cause a continuous reduction of 5,5-dithio-bis-(2-nitrobenzoic acid) (DTNB) to TNB. The product, TNB (5-thio-2-nitrobenzoic acid) is assayed colorimetrically at 412 nm.

Procedure:

Total GSH amount is assayed using the photochemical reduction of DTNB) to TNB. To 0.4 ml of 10 % w/v tissue homogenate, 0.1 ml of 25% aqueous solution of TCA is added. The mixture is vortexed for 2 min and centrifuged at 5000 rpm for 5 min. To the 0.2 ml supernatant, 2 ml of DTNB and 0.8 ml of phosphate buffer was added and absorbance is measured at 412 nm.

7. **Measurement of Thiobarbituric Acid Reactive Substances (TBARS) (Ohkawa et al., 1979)**

   Principle:

   $$LH + L^* + LOO^* \longrightarrow MDA$$

   $$MDA + TBA \longrightarrow PINK\ CLOUR\ COMPLEX$$

   Procedure:

   To 0.2 ml of 10% w/v tissue homogenate, 0.2 ml of 8.1% SDS, 1.5 ml of 20% acetic acid solution and 1.5 ml of 0.8% aqueous solution of TBA is added. The mixture is made upto 4 ml with distilled water and then heated on boiling water bath for 60 mins. After cooling under tap water, 1ml of distilled water and 5 ml of the mixture of n-butanol and pyridine (15:1) are added and vortexed for 2 min. After centrifugation at 2500 g for 10 min, the organic layer was separated and its absorbance at 532 nm was measured.

   Calculation:

   The level of lipid peroxides is expressed in nmol of malonadialdehyde (MDA) using molar extinction coefficient.

C) **Serum biochemical parameters:**

   1. **Quantitative determination of Triglycerides (Cole et al., 1997)**

      Principle:

      $$Triglycerides \underset{}{\overset{LPL}{\rightleftharpoons}} Glycerol + Free\ fatty\ acids$$

      $$Glycerol + ATP \underset{}{\overset{GK}{\rightleftharpoons}} Glycerol\text{-}3\text{-}phosphate + ADP$$

      $$Glycerol\text{-}3\text{-}phosphate + O_2 \underset{}{\overset{GPO}{\rightleftharpoons}} Dihydroxy\ acetone\ phosphate + H_2O_2$$

$$2H_2O_2 + AAP + \text{4-Chloramphenol} \overset{POD}{\rightleftharpoons} \text{Quinoneimine} + HCl + 4H_2O_2$$

Where AAP = Aminoantipyrine

Procedure:

10 μl of serum is mixed with 1 ml reagent and the resulting mixture is incubated at 37°C for 10 min. The absorbance was read within 60 min against blank at 500 nm.

Calculations:

$$\text{Triglycerides (mg/dl)} = \frac{\text{Absorbance of test}}{\text{Absorbance of standard}} \times \text{Concentration of standard (mg/dl)}$$

2. **Quantitative determination of total cholesterol (Richmond, 1973)**
   Principle:

$$\text{Cholesterol ether} + H2O \overset{CHE}{\rightleftharpoons} \text{Cholesterol} + \text{fatty acid}$$

$$\text{Cholesterol} + O2 \overset{CHO}{\rightleftharpoons} \text{Cholesterol} - 3\text{-one} + H_2O_2$$

$$2H_2O_2 + \text{4-Aminoantipyrine} + \text{Phenol} \overset{POD}{\rightleftharpoons} \text{Quinoneimine} + 4H_2O_2$$

Cholesterol and its esters are released from lipoproteins by detergents. Cholesterol esterases hydrolyzes the esters. In subsequent enzymatic oxidation by Cholesterol oxidase, H_2O_2 is formed. This is converted into colored quinoneimine in reaction with 4-Aminoantipyrine and Phenol catalyzed by peroxidase.

Procedure:

10 μl of serum is mixed with 1 ml reagent and the resulting mixture is incubated at 37°C for 10 min. The absorbance is read within 60 min against blank at 500 nm.

Calculations:

$$\text{Total cholesterol (mg/dl)} = \frac{\text{Absorbance of test}}{\text{Absorbance of standard}} \times \text{Concentration of standard (mg/dl)}$$

3. **Quantitative determination of HDL cholesterol (Furedewald et al., 1972)**
   Principle:
   VLDL (very low density lipoproteins) and LDL (low density lipoproteins) are precipitated by addition of phosphotungstic acid and magnesium chloride. After centrifugation the supernatant fluid contaiins the HDL fraction, which is assayed.

   Procedure:
   100 μl of serum is mixed with 100 μl of HDL reagent and the resulting mixture is allowed to stand for 10min at room temperature, mixed and centrifuged. After centrifugation the clear supernatant is separated from the precipitate and cholesterol concentration of the supernatant was determined using cholesterol reagent.

   Calculations:

   $$\text{HDL cholesterol (mg/dl)} = \frac{\text{Absorbance of test}}{\text{Absorbance of standard}} \times \text{Concentration of standard (mg/dl)}$$

   VLDL cholesterol (mg/dl) = Triglyceride/5
   LDL (mg/dl) = Total cholesterol -(HDL+VLDL)

4. **Quantitative determination of Creatinine: (Slot, 1965)**
   Principle:
   Creatinine forms a yellow-orange compound alkaline solution with picric acid. At low picric acid concentration a precipitation of proteins does not take place. The concentration of dyestuff formed over a certain reaction time is the measure of creatinine concentration.

   As a result of rapid reaction between creatinine and picric acid, later secondary reactions do not cause interference. This method thus distinguishes itself by its high specificity.

Procedure:

20 μl of serum is mixed with 1 ml of picric acid reagent. The absorbance of test and standard is read immediately and after 5 minutes against 500 nm.

Calculations:

Creatinine conc. (mg/dl)= (As2-As1/Ast2-Ast1) $\times$ 88.4 (μmol/l).

Where,

As1: Initial O.D of test

As2: Final O.D of test

Ast1: Initial O.D of standard

Ast2: Final O.D of standard

5. **Quantitative Determination of Urea (Talke and Schubert, 1965)**

Principle:

Urea condenses with O-phthaldehyde and naphthyl ethylene diamine (NED) to form colored complex. The rate of formation of this complex is directly proportional to the urea concentraion in the sample and is measured in an initial rate mode at 500 nm.

Procedure:

30μl of serum is mixed with 1 ml urea reagent. The absorbance of test and standard is read immediately and after 1 minute against 500 nm.

Calculations:

Urea conc (mg/dl) = (As2-As1/Ast2-Ast1) $\times$ 50

Where,

As1: Initial O.D of test

As2: Final O.D of test

Ast1: Initial O.D of standard

Ast2: Final O.D of standard

References:

1. Rajadurai, M., and P. Stanely Mainzen Prince. "Preventive effect of naringin on lipid peroxides and antioxidants in isoproterenol-induced cardiotoxicity in Wistar rats: biochemical and histopathological evidences." Toxicology 228.2-3 (2006): 259-268.

2. Bergmeyer, H. U., M. Horder, and R. Rej. "Approved Recommendation (1985) on IFCC methods for the measurement of catalytic concentration of enzymes. 3. IFCC method for alanine aminotransferase (L-alanine-2-oxoglutarate aminotransferase, EC-2612)." Journal of Clinical Chemistry and Clinical Biochemistry 24.7 (1986): 481-495.

3. Amador, Elias, Lionel E. Dorfman, and Warren EC Wacker. "Serum lactic dehydrogenase activity: an analytical assessment of current assays." Clinical Chemistry 9.4 (1963): 391-399.

4. Roth Jr, Eugene F., and Harriet S. Gilbert. "The pyrogallol assay for superoxide dismutase: absence of a glutathione artifact." Analytical biochemistry 137.1 (1984): 50-53.

ANTI-DIARROHEAL SCREENING (*in-vivo* and *in-vitro*) METHODS

INTRODUCTION:

Diarrhoea is characterized by alteration in secretion, absorption of water and electrolytes and alteration in motility of gastrointestinal tract. The pathophysiology includes change in active ion transport by either decreased sodium absorption or increased chloride secretion; change in intestinal motility; increase in luminal osmolarity and increase in tissue hydrostatic pressure. These mechanisms have been related to four broad clinical diarrhoeal groups: secretory, osmotic, exudative, and altered intestinal transit (Dipiro et al., 2010).

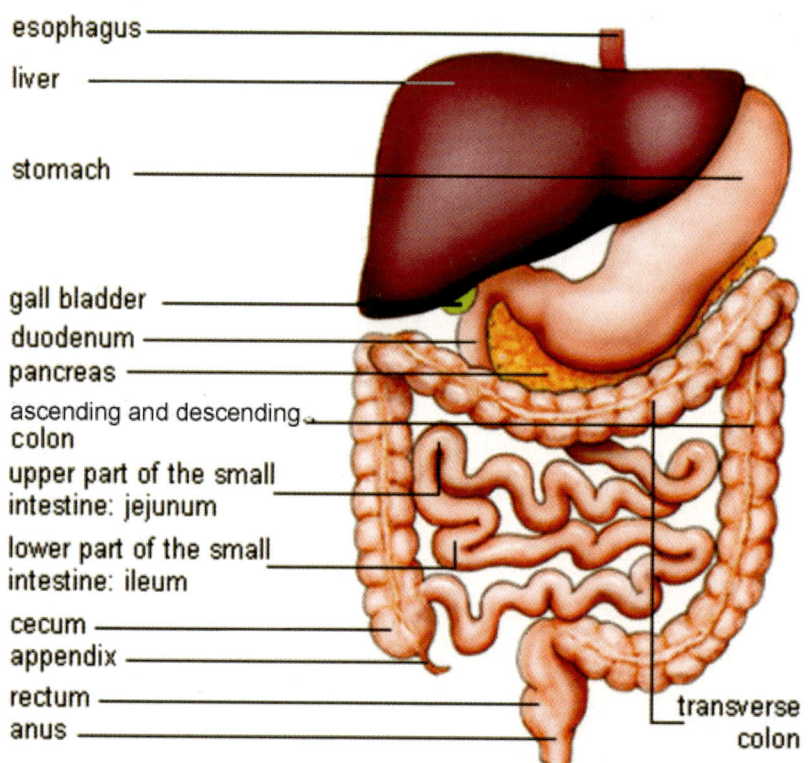

Fig. 12.1: Human gastrointestinal tract (Dipiro et al., 2010).

Water and electrolytes are absorbed as well as secreted in the intestine. Jejunum allows freely permeable salt and water which are passively absorbed secondary to absorption of nutrients (glucose, amino acids, etc). In the ileum and colon, active $Na^+K^+ATPase$ mediated salt absorption occurs, primarily in the mature cells lining villous tips. In addition, glucose facilitated Na^+ absorption takes place in the ileum by sodium glucose co-transporter. This mechanism remains intact even in severe diarrhoea. The osmotic load of luminal contents plays an important role in determining final stool water volume. When non absorbable solutes are present and in disaccharide deficiency (which occurs during starvation), the stool water is increased. Inhibition of $Na^+K^+ATPase$ and structural damage to mucosal cell (by Rotavirus) causes diarrhorea by reducing absorption. Intracellular cyclic nucleotides are important regulators of absorptive and secretory processes. Stimuli enhancing cAMP or cGMP cause net loss of salt and water, both by inhibiting NaCl absorption in villous cells and by promoting anion secretion (Na^+ accompanies) in the crypt cells which are primarily secretory (James et al., 1972).

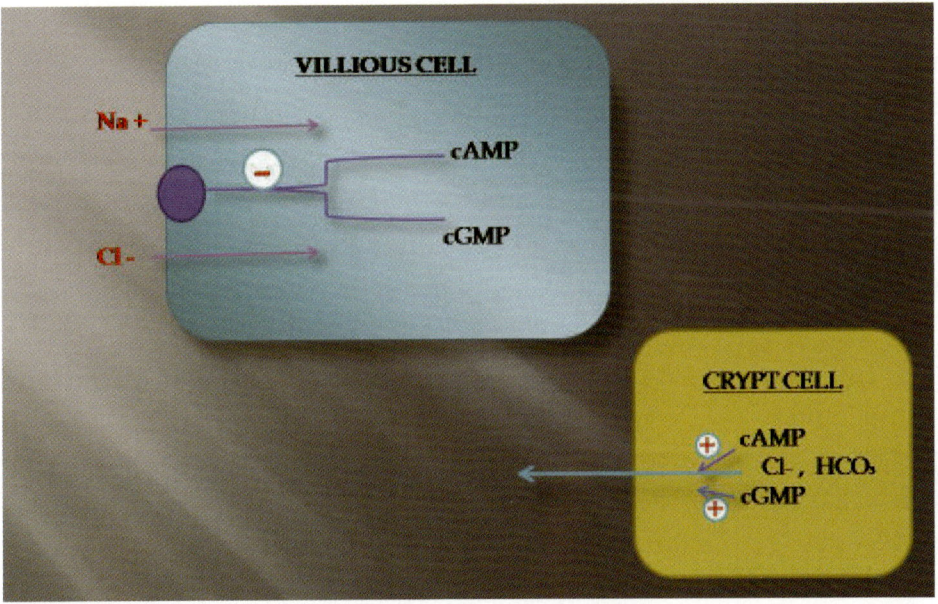

Fig. 12.2: Action of cyclic nucleotides on electrolyte transport of intestinal mucosal cells
(James et al., 1972).

Secretory diarrhoea occurs when a stimulating substance either increases secretion or decreases absorption of large amounts of water and electrolytes. Substances that cause excess secretion include vasoactive intestinal peptide (VIP) from a pancreatic tumor, unabsorbed dietary fat, laxatives, hormones (such as secretin), bacterial toxins and excessive bile salts. Many of these agents stimulate intracellular cyclic adenosine monophosphate and inhibit Na^+K^+-ATPase leading to increased secretion. Also, many of these mediators inhibit ion absorption simultaneously. Poorly absorbed substances retain intestinal fluids, resulting in osmotic diarrhoea. This process occurs with malabsorption syndromes, lactose intolerance, administration of divalent ions (e.g., magnesium containing antacids) or consumption of poorly soluble carbohydrate like lactulose. Inflammatory diseases of the gastrointestinal tract discharge mucus, serum proteins and blood into the gut. Sometimes bowel movements consist only of mucus, exudate and blood. Exudative diarrhoea probably affects other absorptive, secretory, or motility functions to account for the large stool volume associated with this disorder.

Altered intestinal motility produces diarrhoea by three mechanisms: reduction of contact time in the small intestine, premature emptying of the colon, and bacterial overgrowth. Chyme must be exposed to intestinal epithelium for a sufficient time period to enable normal absorption and secretion processes to occur. Decrease in this contact time results in diarrhoea. Intestinal resection or bypass surgery and drugs (such as metoclopramide) cause this type of diarrhoea. On the other hand, an increased time of exposure allows fecal bacteria overgrowth. A characteristic small intestine diarrhoeal pattern is rapid, small, coupling bursts of waves. These waves are inefficient, do not allow absorption, and rapidly dump chyme into the colon. Once in the colon, chyme exceeds the colonic capability to absorb water.

Table 12.1: Infectious causes of acute diarrhoea with nausea and vomiting (Jones and farthings 2004)

Agent	Incubation	Duration	Age
Staphylococcus aureus	30 min - 8 hrs usually 2 - 4 hrs	< 24 hrs	All ages
Rotavirus	15 - 77 hrs usually 24 - 48 hrs	5 - 7 days	3 - 15 months
Enteric adenovirus	15 – 77 hrs usually 24 - 48 hrs	5 - 12 days	< 2 years
Norwalk virus	15 - 77 hrs usually 24 - 48 hrs	1 - 2 days	Older children and adults
Calcivirus	15 - 77 hrs usually 24 - 48 hrs	1 - 2 days	All ages
Astrovirus	15 - 77 hrs usually 24 - 48 hrs	2 - 3 days	Pediatric

Table 12.2: Infectious causes of secretory diarrhoea

Agent	Incubation	Duration	Source
Vibrio cholera	1-5 days	1-6 days peak stool volume within 24 hr	Fecal-oral; contaminated water shellfish
Enterotoxigenic E. Coli (ETEC)	6-48 hrs	5-10 days	Food
C. perfringens	6-24 hrs	24 hrs	Meats
Bacillus cereus	6-24 hrs	< 24 hrs	Improperly stored cooked foods (rice, pasta, sauces, meat)
Giardia lamblia	3-25 days median 7 days	2-3 months	Water, person-person
Cryptosporidium parvum	2-28 days median 7 days	10 days	Water, food, person-person
Cyclospora	1-11 days median 7 days	5 days (relapses)	Water, food
Dientomoeba fragilis	5-8 days	1-2 weeks	E. vermicularis (pinworm)

Table 12.3: Infectious causes of inflammatory diarrhoea

Agent	Incubation	Duration	Source
Nontyphoidal *Salmonella*	6 hrs - 10 days usually 6-48 hrs	3 days (1 - 14 days)	Eggs, meat, poultry, dairy
Shigella	12 hrs - 16 days usually 2-4 days	3 days (1 - 14 days)	Salads, eggs, potato, poultry
Campylobacter	2-10 days usually 2 - 5 days	7 days (2 - 30 days)	Chicken, milk, person-person
E. coli	1 - 10 days usually 3 - 4 days	- 7 days (1->31 days)	Food, water person-person
Enteroinvasive E. coli	Variable	5 - 7 days	Food or water

Agent	Incubation	Duration	Source
C. difficile	Several days after starting, 8 weeks after stopping	Prolonged	High rate asymptomatic carriage (nosocomial)
E. histolytica	1 - 2 weeks	Variable	Food or water
Yersinia enterocolitica	1 - 10 days usually 4 - 6 days	1 - 3 weeks	meat or dairy

Management of diarrhoea includes non pharmacological management and pharmacological management.

Non pharmacologic management includes Dietary management, Water and electrolyte replacement and Oral rehydration salt (ORS) or homemade rehydration solution.

Pharmacologic management includes Antimotility agents (Loperamide, Diphenoxylate, Codeine); Adsorbents (Polycarbophil, Ispaghula, Psyllium, Methyl cellulose); Antisecretory agents (Bismuth subsalicylate, Sulfasalazine, Mesalazine); Antimicrobials (Cotrimoxazole, Ciprofloxacin, Ampicillin, Metronidazole) and Miscellaneous products (Lactobacillus preparations, lactase enzyme).

Dietary management is a first priority in the treatment of diarrhoea. Rehydration and maintenance of water and electrolytes are primary treatment goals until the diarrhoeal episode ends. For this reason, oral rehydration salts (ORS) are strongly recommended. ORS is absorbed in the small intestine and replaces the water and electrolytes lost in the feces (Chandan S., 2005).

Antimotility agents like loperamide is effective at reducing the duration of diarrhoea. Codeine is used in the treatment of diarrhoea to slow down peristalsis and the passage of fecal material through the bowels (Finkel et al., 2005).

SCREENING METHODS FOR EVALUATION OF ANTIDIARRHOEAL ACTIVITY

Antidiarrhoeal potential of test extract is evaluated using various animal models which are based on the fact that diarrhoea is related to excess secretion of water and electrolytes, decreased absorption and increased motility of gastrointestinal tract. Onset of diarrhoeal action, number and weight of stools are measured correctly. Among all models castor oil induced diarrhoea model is widely used by researchers. Motility of gastrointestinal tract is measured by using charcoal meal test. These models help to investigate pharmacological effect and possible mechanism of action of test drug.

CASTOR OIL INDUCED DIARRHOEA MODEL

This *in-vivo* model is a widely used by researchers to evaluate antidiarrhoeal effect. Castor oil is easily available and parameters are simple to evaluate. Several mechanisms have been previously proposed to explain the diarrhoeal effect of castor oil including inhibition of intestinal Na^+K^+ ATPase activity to reduce normal fluid absorption, activation of adenyle cyclase or mucosal cAMP mediated active secretion, stimulation of prostaglandin formation, platelet activating factor and recently nitric oxide has been claimed to contribute to the diarrhoeal effect of castor oil (Alam et al., 2008). Ricinoleic acid produces changes in the transport of water and electrolytes resulting in a hypersecretory response. In addition to hypersecretion, ricinoleic acid sensitizes the intramural neurons of the gut. Castor oil produces secretory type diarrhoea.

Mice weighing between 25-30 g are used for the study. Mice are fasted overnight prior to experiment (with free access to water). Mice are divided into three groups Control group, positive control group and test group. All drugs are given by oral route with the help of feeding needle. Group I receives normal saline (10 ml/Kg) and serves as control group. Group II receives standard drug loperamide (4 mg/Kg) and serves as positive control group. Group III receives test drug and serves as test group. 30 min after administration of last dose all the animals are treated with castor oil (10 ml/Kg). Observations for defecation is continued on pre-weighed (M_0) filter paper placed beneath the individual perforated observation cages. This paper is replaced every hour. The used filter paper is reweighed (M_1) if it had wet feces. The fresh weight of feces is evaluated as $(M_1 - M_0)$ gm. Finally, the filter paper is exposed in the laboratory to dry over a period of 14 h and is reweighed again (M_2). The water content of the feces is calculated as $(M_2 - M_1)$ gm.

For evaluation of antidiarrhoeal activity each mouse is placed in individual metabolic cage with floor lined by blotting paper. Each mouse is observed for period of four hours. Onset of diarrhoeal action, number of wet stools, total number of stools, weight of wet stools, total weight of stools is observed. For determination of evacuation index (EI) of each group, numerical scores are assigned to the stools (Salud et al., 2005).

Scores are given as:
0= no stool, 1= solid stool, 2= semisolid stool and 3= liquid stool.

EI is calculated by using formula-
EI = 1(solid stools) + 2(semisolid stools) + 3(liquid stools).

Parameters like onset of action, number and weight of wet stools, total weight of stools and evacuation index helps to correlate between test and control groups. Delayed onset of action by test groups signifies decreased action of castor oil. Decreased weight and number of wet stools signifies inhibition of hypersecretory response by test drugs (Ching et al., 2009).

MAGNESIUM SULPHATE INDUCED DIARRHOEA MODEL

Magnesium sulphate has been reported to induce diarrhoea (dose 2 gm/kg) by increasing the volume of intestinal content through prevention of reabsorption of water. It has also been reported that it promotes the liberation of cholecystokinin from the duodenal mucosa, which increases the secretion and motility of small intestine and thereby prevents the reabsorption of sodium chloride and water (Uddin et al 2005).

Similar protocol and evaluation as that of castor oil induced diarrhoea model is followed in this model. Magnesium sulphate (2 gm/kg, p.o) is used to induce diarrhoea instead of castor oil (Uddin et al., 2005). Mice weighing between 25-30 g are used for the study. Mice are fasted overnight prior to experiment (with free access to water). Mice are divided into three groups Control group, positive control group and test group. All drugs are given by oral route with the help of feeding needle. Group I receives normal saline (10 ml/Kg) and serves as control group. Group II receives standard drug loperamide (4 mg/Kg) and serves as positive control group. Group III receives test drug and serves as test group. 30 min after administration of last dose all the animals are treated with magnesium sulphate (2 gm/kg). Observations for defecation continued on pre-weighed (M_0) filter paper placed beneath the individual perforated observation cages. This paper is replaced every hour. The used filter paper is reweighed (M_1) if it had wet feces. The fresh weight of feces is evaluated as ($M_1 - M_0$) g. Finally, the filter paper is exposed in the laboratory to dry over a period of 14 h and was reweighed again (M_2). The water content of the feces is calculated as ($M_2 - M_1$) gm.

Each mouse is placed in individual metabolic cage with floor lined by blotting paper. Each mouse is observed for period of four hours. Onset of diarrhoeal action, number of wet stools, total number of stools, weight of wet stools, total weight of stools is observed. For determination of evacuation index (EI) of each group, numerical scores are assigned to the stools.

Scores are given as:
0= no stool, 1= solid stool, 2= semisolid stool and 3= liquid stool.

EI is calculated by using formula -
EI = 1 (solid stools) + 2 (semisolid stools) + 3 (liquid stools).

SMALL INTESTINAL TRANSIT STUDY

Small intestinal transit is an *in vivo* method studied by using charcoal meal test. Charcoal meal is mixture of 3% activated charcoal into 10% gum acacia. This test helps us to study effect of test extracts on gastrointestinal motility which is calculated by percent inhibition of charcoal meal movement by test groups compared with normal group.

This method is adopted to study the effect of extract on the gastrointestinal transit in mice. Mice weighing between 25-30 g are used for the study. Mice are fasted overnight prior to experiment (with free access to water). Mice are divided into three groups control group, positive control group and test group. All drugs are given by oral route with the help of feeding needle. Group I receives normal saline (10 ml/Kg) and serves as control group. Group II receives standard drug loperamide (4 mg/Kg) and serves as positive control group. Group III receives test drug and serves as test group. 30 min after administration of last dose all the animals are treated with magnesium sulphate (2 gm/kg). 30 min after administration of last dose mice of each group are fed with 1 ml of charcoal meal. 30 min after administration of charcoal meal mice of each group are sacrificed. Abdomen is opened. Length of small intestine from pyloric sphincter to caecum as well as distance travelled by charcoal meal is measured (Nwafor et al., 2000).

Charcoal movement in small intestine is expressed in percentage by a formula-
% movement of charcoal meal = (Distance travelled by charcoal head) / (Total length of small intestine) × 100

EFFECTS ON ISOLATED RABBITS ILEUM

This *in-vitro* method has been used for many purposes, such as the study of the effects of adrenaline on the lower segments causing contraction and on the segments of the upper end causing relaxation. The model is used as a basic screening procedure for spasmolytic activity, whereby an anti-acetylcholine or anticarbachol effect indicates antimuscarinic activity and an anti- barium chloride effect indicates a musculotropic effect. In addition to the isolated ileum, other parts of the gut such as the isolated duodenum and colon have been used widely.

The method has been used for many purposes, such as the study on the effects of adrenaline on the lower segments causing contraction and on the segments of the upper end causing relaxation. The model is used as a basic screening procedure for anti-muscarinic activity where an anti-acetylcholine or anti-carbachol effect is studied.

Adult male rabbit weighing 1.5 kg is starved for 12 hours before the experiment. Thereafter it is humanely sacrificed. Abdomen is opened out and segments of ileum about 2 centimeters are cut and washed. All segments are mounted in a 10-ml tissue organ tube filled with Tyrode's solution of composition (mM): NaCl (136.8), KCl (2.7), $CaCl_2$ (1.3), $NaHCO_3$ (11.9), $MgCl_2$ (0.5), Na_2PO_4 (0.45) and glucose (5.5).

Organ tube is continuously aerated with Carbogen (95% Oxygen and 5% CO_2) and maintained at a temperature of 37 (±1°C). 1 gram of preload is applied to each segments of ileum. Each segment is equilibrated for 30 min. before addition of any drug. Intestinal contractions are recorded using isotonic frontal writing lever on digital Sherrington rotating drum.

Effect of serial addition of acetylcholine, standard drug and test drug are recorded on student kymograph. Further effects of serial addition of drugs are recorded in presence of fixed concentration of acetylcholine. Contact time of 1 min. for every dose addition is followed by three successive washing periods. Resting period of 10 min. is allowed before next addition (Suleiman et al., 2008).

References:

1. Alam, M. A., Akter, R., Subhan, N,M., Rahman, M., Majumder, M. M., Nahar, L., Sarker, S.D, 2008. Antidiarrhoeal property of the hydroethanolic extract of the flowering tops of Anthocephalus cadamba, Brazilian J Pharmacog. 18(2), 155-159.

2. Chandan, S. K. Quintessence and medicinal pharmacology, 2005, 3rd ed. New central book agency Pvt. Ltd, Kolkatta (India), pp. 378-380.

3. Ching, F.P., Okpo, S.D., Falodun, A. and Omogbai S. 2009. Antidiarrhoeal activity of chromatographic fractions of Stereospermum kunthianum cham sandrine Petit (Bignoniaceae) Stem Bark, Tropical Journal of Pharmaceutical Research 8(6), 515-519.

4. Dipiro, J.T., Talbert, R.L., Tee, G.C., Matzeke, G.R., Wells, B.G., Posey, L.M., 2008, Pharmacotherapy- A Pathophysiologic Approach, 6th ed., 2008, Mc Graw Hill Publications, pp. 677-692.

5. Finkel, R., Lippincott's illustrated reviews, Pharmacology, 4th ed., 2005. Wollters Kluwer Ind. Pvt. Ltd, New Delhi (India), pp.338-340.

6. James, W.P.T., Drasar, B.S., Miller, C., 1972. Physiological mechanism and pathogenesis of weanling diarrhea. American Journal of Clinical Nutrition 25, 564-571.

7. Jones, A.C and Farthing, M. J. G, 2004. Management of infectious diarrhea Gut. 53, 296-305.

8. Nwafor, P.A., Okwuasaba, F.K., Binda, L.G., 2000. Antidiarrhoeal and antiulcerogenic effects of Asparagus pubescens root in rats. J. Ethnopharmacol. 72, 421-427.

9. Salud, P.G., Cuauhtemoc, P.G., Zavala, M.A S., 2005. A study of the antidiarrhoeal properties of Loeselia mexicana on mice and rats. Phytomedicine 12, 670-674.

10. Suleiman, M.M., Dzenda, T., Sani, C.A., 2008. Antidiarrhoeal activity of the methanol stem-bark extract of Annonasenegalensis Pres. (Annonaceae). J. Ethnopharmacol. 116, 125-130.

11. Uddin, S.J., Shilpi, J.A., Alam, S.M.S., Alamgir, M., Rahman, M.T., Sarker, S.D., 2005. Antidiarrhoeal activity of methanol extract of the barks of Xylocarpus miluccensis in castor oil and magnesium sulphate induced diarrhoea models in mice. J. Ethnopharmacol. 101, 139-149.

12. Wendel, G.H., Maria, A.O.M., Guzman, J.A., Giordano, O., Plezer, L.E., 2008. Antidiarrhoeal activity of dehydroleucodine isolated from Artemisia douglasiana. Fitoterapia 79, 1-5.

13 BIOSTATISTICAL METHODS IN PRE-CLINICAL RESEARCH

INTRODUCTION

This chapter aims to provide basic knowledge of biostatistics and applications to researchers in Pre-clinical study and also to help them in solving their problems. This chapter contains relevant examples to help to clarify the concepts. It explains how to choose an appropriate statistical analysis for various pre-clinical experimental data. The computational steps and interpretation of the findings are also given. This chapter will help the researchers to choose appropriate statistical techniques for a proper analysis of their research data and draw valid conclusions.

Statistics is an important tool in pharmacological research that is used to summarize experimental data in terms of descriptive statistical measures such as central tendency, (mean or median), variance (standard deviation, standard error of the mean) and confidence interval. Descriptive statistics particularly enables conduct of hypothesis testing, and revolve around certain assumptions regarding the nature of data. These assumptions form the basis of several statistical tests including the student's t-test, paired t-test, chi-square analysis, wilcoxon signed-rank test, etc.

Observations from biological laboratory experiments, clinical trials, and health surveys always carry some amount of uncertainty. In many cases, especially for the laboratory experiments, it is inevitable to just ignore these uncertainties due to large variation in observations. Statistical tools may be useful in abolishing these uncertainties while filtering out noise from the available data. Scientific experiments present an opportunity to generate rich and valuable data, which need to be validated through statistical tools. In this course, we will discuss about different statistical tools required to:
i)   Analyze our observations,

ii) Design new experiments,

iii) Integrate large number of observations in single unified model.

The field of statistics is divided into two major divisions: descriptive and inferential. Each of two segments is important, offering different techniques that accomplish different objectives. Descriptive statistics describe what is going on in a population or data set. Inferential statistics, in contrast, allow researchers to take findings from a sample group and generalize them to a larger population.

The two types of statistics have some important differences as summarized below:

1) Descriptive Statistics
Descriptive statistics is the type of statistics that probably springs to most people's minds when they hear the word "statistics". In this branch of statistics, the goal is to describe data. Numerical measures are used to present the features of a data-set. Following are the measures used to infer the characteristics of data, using descriptive statistics.

The average or measure of the center of a data is indicated by mean and the spread of a data set can be measured with standard deviation. These measures are important and useful because they allow researchers to see patterns with reference to data, and thus make sense of the available data. Descriptive statistics can only be used to describe the population or data set under study, the results cannot be generalized to any other group or population.

Types of Descriptive Statistics
There are two kinds of descriptive statistics that pre-clinical researchers use: Measures of central tendency capture general trends within the data and are calculated and expressed as the mean, median, and mode. A mean tells us the mathematical average of all of a data set.

Arithmetic mean
One of the objectives of the analysis of data is to get one single value which can describe characteristics of the entire mass of a data-set which can be considered as representative of the entire distribution. A value satisfying this criterion is a central value or an "average". Let $x_1, x_2, \ldots, x_n$ be 'n' observations on a random variable x, then the arithmetic mean, denoted by $\bar{x}$, is calculated as

$$\bar{x} = \frac{Sum\ of\ the\ observations}{Number\ of\ observations}$$

i.e. $\bar{x} = \dfrac{\sum\limits_{i=1}^{n} x_i}{n}$.

Example 1: Calculate arithmetic mean for the following data:

Serial number	1	2	3	4	5	6
Body weights of Wistar rats (in gms)	180	200	175	180	174	192

Here number of observations, n=6.

$\sum_{1}^{6} x = 180 + 200 + \ldots + 192 = 1101$ and $\bar{x} = \dfrac{\sum\limits_{i=1}^{n} x_i}{n} = \dfrac{1101}{6} = 183.5.$

Therefore average body weights of 6 rats is 183.5 gms.

Measures of Dispersion:

In addition to averages, some additional information about the variation of items is required to know the extent to which the values vary from one another and from central value. Measures of spread or scatter of the data is called a **measure of variation or dispersion.** The measures of dispersion determine the extent of variation in the data by, which, some steps can be taken to control the variability.

Variance and standard deviation:

A measure of dispersion, which takes into account all the observations in the data, is variance or standard deviation. Variance is defined as the arithmetic mean of the squares of the deviation of the observations from their arithmetic mean. It is denoted by σ^2, positive square root of the variance is called standard deviation and is denoted by σ.

Let $x_1, x_2, x_3 \ldots \ldots x_n$ be a set of observations on random variable x, then standard deviation of x is defined as $\sigma = \sqrt{\dfrac{\sum\limits_{i=1}^{n} (x_i - \bar{x})^2}{n}}$ which can also be written as

$$\sigma = \sqrt{\frac{\sum\limits_{i=1}^{n} x^2}{n} - \bar{x}^2} \; .$$

Example 2: Calculate standard deviation and variance for the following data:

Serial number	1	2	3	4	5	6
Body weights of Wistar rats (in gms)	180	200	175	180	174	192

Here number of observations is n=6.

$\sum_{1}^{6} x = 180 + 200 + \ldots + 192 = 1101$ and $\bar{x} = \dfrac{\sum\limits_{i=1}^{n} x_i}{n} = \dfrac{1101}{6} = 183.5$.

Therefore average body weights of 6 rats are 183.5 gms.

$\sum_{1}^{6} x^2 = 180^2 + 200^2 + \ldots + 192^2 = 202{,}565$

$$\sigma = \sqrt{\frac{\sum\limits_{i=1}^{n} x^2}{n} - \bar{x}^2} = \sqrt{\frac{202{,}565}{6} - 183.5^2} = \sqrt{33760.8333 - 33672.25} = \sqrt{88.5833} = 9.4118 \, .$$

$\sigma^2 = 88.5833$.

The variation of body weights of wistar rats from average 183.5 gms is 88.5833 gms.

2) Inferential Statistics

Inferential statistics are produced through complex mathematical calculations that allow scientists to infer trends about a larger population based on a study of a sample taken from it. Researchers use inferential statistics to examine the relationships between variables within a sample and then make conclusions or predictions about how those variables will relate to a larger population. It is usually impossible to examine each member of the population individually. So researchers choose a representative subset of the population, called a statistical sample, and from this analysis, they are able to comment on the nature of population from which the sample is drawn. There are two major divisions of inferential statistics:

- A confidence interval which gives a range of values for an unknown parameter of the population by measuring a statistical sample. This is expressed in terms of an interval and the degree of confidence that the parameter is within the interval.

- Tests of significance or hypothesis testing where researchers make a claim about the population by analyzing a statistical sample. By design, there is some uncertainty in this process. This can be expressed in terms of a level of significance.

Techniques that researchers use to examine the relationships between variables, and thereby to create inferential statistics, includes, Analysis of variance (ANOVA). When conducting research using inferential statistics, researchers conduct a test of significance to determine whether they can generalize their results to a larger population. Common tests of significance include the chi-square and t-test. These tells researchers the probability that the results of their analysis of the sample are representative of the population as a whole.

Descriptive vs. Inferential Statistics

Although descriptive statistics is helpful in learning things such as the spread and center of the data, nothing in descriptive statistics can be used to make any generalizations. In descriptive statistics, measurements such as the mean and standard deviation are stated as exact numbers.

Even though inferential statistics uses some similar calculations such as the mean and standard deviation, the focus is different for inferential statistics. Inferential statistics start with a sample and then generalizes to a population. This information about a population is not stated as a number, Instead, researchers express these parameters as a range of potential numbers along with a degrees of confidence.

Definitions for Confidence interval:

In statistics a confidence interval is a type of interval estimate of a population parameter and is used to indicate the reliability of an estimate .It is an observed interval in principle different from sample to sample that frequently includes the parameter of interest if the experiment is repeated, how frequently the observed interval contains the parameter is determined by the confidence level or confidence coefficient. The **confidence level** is the frequency (i.e., the proportion) of possible confidence intervals that contain the true value of their corresponding parameter. Confidence intervals consist of a range of values (interval) that act as good estimates of the unknown **population parameter.** However, the interval computed from a particular sample does not necessarily include the true value of the parameter.

Since the observed data are random samples from the true population, the confidence interval obtained from the data is also random. If a corresponding hypothesis test is performed, the confidence level is the complement of the level of significance; for example, a 95% confidence interval reflects a significance level of 0.05. If it is hypothesized that a true parameter value is 0 but the 95% confidence interval does not contain 0, then the estimate is significantly different from zero at the 5% significance level. The desired level of confidence is set by the researcher (not determined by data). Most commonly, the 95% confidence level is used. However, other confidence levels can be used, for example, 90% and 99%.

Testing of Hypothesis (Parametric tests):

Sometimes we require to test certain statements (hypothesis) about population parameters. This is called testing of hypothesis. In other words, a hypothesis is a conclusion which is tentatively drawn on logical basis. For example, the average RBC count of Human blood is 5.5 millions per cubic millimeter, can be classified as a hypothesis which can be measured and assessed. When dealing with a hypothesis test we have to formulate our initial research hypothesis into two statements which can be evaluated as null and alternative hypothesis.

Statistical hypothesis: It is tentative conclusion that specifies the properties of a distribution of a random variable. These properties generally refer to parameters of the population and are hypothetical values with which the values of statistic derived from a sample are compared in order to find the difference between statistic and corresponding parameter. In other words, statistical hypothesis is some assumption or statement, which may or may not be true, about a population or about the probability distribution characterizing the given population, which we want to test on the basis of the evidence from a random sample.

Test of significance: The testing of hypothesis is a procedure that helps us to ascertain the likelihood of hypothesized population parameter being correct by making use of the sample statistic. In other words, it is a process of test of significance which concerns with the testing of some hypothesis regarding a parameter of the population on the basis of statistic from the sample.

In testing of hypothesis, a statistic is computed from a sample drawn from the parent population and on the basis of this statistic, it is observed whether the sample so drawn has come from the corresponding population parameter due to sampling fluctuations. The test of hypothesis discloses the fact whether the difference between sample statistic and the corresponding hypothetical population parameter is significant or not significant. Thus the test of hypothesis is also known as the **test of significance.**

Procedure for testing of Hypothesis

The following are the steps involved in testing of hypothesis:

Setting up of hypothesis. There are two types of hypothesis:

i)   **Null hypothesis**

ii) **Alternative hypothesis**

Null hypothesis: The statistical hypothesis that is set up for testing a hypothesis is known as null hypothesis. The null hypothesis test is set up in testing a statistical hypothesis only to decide whether to accept or reject the null hypothesis. It asserts that there is no difference between the sample statistic and population parameter and whatever difference exists, is attributable to sampling errors. Null hypothesis is usually denoted by H_0. e.g. In vitamin C tablet if content of vitamin C claimed on label is 500 mg, it can be considered as null hypothesis H_0.

Alternative hypothesis: The negation of null hypothesis is called the alternative hypothesis. In other words, any hypothesis which is not a null hypothesis is called an alternative hypothesis. It is always denoted by H_1. It is set in such a way that the rejection of null hypothesis implies the acceptance of alternative hypothesis. e.g. On assay in quality control unit if the content and vitamin C is found to be 470 mg, it can be considered as alternative hypothesis H_1.

Types of Errors in hypothesis Testing: There is every chance that a decision regarding a null hypothesis may be correct. There are two types of errors:

a)   **Type I error:** It is the error of rejecting null hypothesis H_0, when it is true. When a null hypothesis is true, but the difference is significant and the hypothesis is rejected, then a **Type I error** is made. **The probability of making a** type I error is **denoted by α, the level of significance.** In order to control the type I error, the probability of type I error is fixed at a certain level of significance α. **The probability of making a correct decision then will be $(1-\alpha)$.**

b)   **Type II error:** It is the error of accepting the null hypothesis H_0 when it is false. In other words, when a null hypothesis is false, but the difference is insignificant and the hypothesis is accepted, a type II error is made. **The probability of making a type II error is denoted by β.**

Level of Significance (l.o.s): The level of significance represents the amount of risk that a researchers will accept when making a decision. Whenever research is undertaken, we will always have the probability that the data is subject to chance. If the level of significance is α then it indicates that there could be α % error in conclusion. It represents the amount of error associated with rejecting the null hypothesis when it is true.

Statistical definition: The level of significance is the maximum probability of making a type I error and it is denoted by α, i.e., P [Rejecting H_0, when H_0 is true]$=\alpha$. The probability of making a correct decision is then $(1-\alpha)$. The best value for fixing the level of significance depends on the seriousness of the results of the types of error. The commonly used level of significance in practice are 5% (0.05) and 1% (0.01). If we use 5% level of significance ($\alpha = 0.05$), we shall mean that the probability of making type I error is 0.05 or 5% i.e. **P [Rejecting H_0 when H_0 is true] = 0.05.** This means that there is a probability of making 5 out of 100 (or making 1 out of 20) type I error. This also means that we are 95% confident that a correct decision has been made. Similarly 1% level of significance ($\alpha =0.01$) means that there is a probability of making 1 error out of 100. It is important to note that if no **level of significance is given, then we always take $\alpha=0.05$.**

Interpretation: If an analyst states that the results are significant at the 5% level then what they are saying is that there is a 5% probability that the sample data values collected have occurred by chance. An alternative view is to use the concept of a confidence interval. In this case we can observe that we are 95% confident that the results have not occurred by chance.

P - value: The p-value is used to decide on accepting or rejecting H_0. The p-value represents the probability of the calculated random sample test statistic being this extreme if the null hypothesis is true. This p-value can then be compared to the chosen significance level to make a decision between accepting or rejecting the null hypothesis. Thus, p-value is the level of marginal significance within a statistical hypothesis test representing the probability of the occurrence of a given event. The p-value is used as an alternative to rejection points to provide the smallest level of significance at which the null hypothesis would be rejected. A smaller p-value means that there is stronger evidence in favor of the alternative hypothesis. This p-value can then be compared to the chosen significance level to make a decision between accepting or rejecting null hypothesis.

Interpretation: Although theoretically one can compute p-value, however now-a-days it is derive from software. If $p < \alpha$, $(\alpha = 0.05)$ then we would reject the null hypothesis H_0 and accept the alternative hypothesis H_1 Vice-versa.

Critical Statistic/Value: A different approach for using the p-value is to calculate the test statistic and compare the value with a critical test statistic estimate from an appropriate statistical table (reference table). The critical value for a hypothesis test is a limit at which the value of the sample test statistic is judged to be such that the null hypothesis may be rejected. The value of the critical test statistic will depend upon the following factors: (i) significance level for z-test problems (refer to large sample test), and (ii) the significance level and number of degrees of freedom for the problems discussed in t, chi-square and F tests etc below. This critical test statistic can then be compared with the calculated test statistic to make a decision between accepting and rejecting the null hypothesis. Critical values for any statistical test can be obtained from alternative hypothesis.

Interpretation: If test statistic > critical test statistic then we would reject the null hypothesis and accept the alternative hypothesis.

Procedure for testing of hypothesis:
The procedure for testing of hypothesis is as follows:
1. Set up the null hypothesis H_0 and alternative hypothesis H_1.
2. Specify the level of significance α.
3. Check whether sample size is large or small.
4. Write down sample data in brief.
5. Identify the test statistics suitable for the test and find its value for the given sample data under null hypothesis H_0.
6. Find critical value at α % level of significance.
7. Compare the critical value of test statistics for given data with critical value in reference table. If calculated value of test statistics is greater than or equal to critical value, then reject H_0 and accept H_1, if calculated value of test statistics is less than critical value (table value), then we accept H_0.
8. Draw conclusion according to above rules.

After having an idea of various concepts of testing of hypothesis, the applications of the said procedure are considered, all of which may be termed as test of significance. The purpose of test of significance is to aid the clinician, the researchers or the administrator in reaching a decision concerning a population by examining only a sample from the population. As the sample must be random to reach a reliable and valid decision.

Large sample test: In large sample test sample size is greater than 30 (n>30). In large sample test the test statistic is standard normal varaite.

One sample problems for testing Mean:

Let x be a normal variable with unknown mean μ and known variance σ^2. Let $x_1, x_2, \ldots, x_n$ be a random sample drawn from this population then we have to test whether population mean has a specified value μ_0 *(mean of data) or* not.

Test Procedure: Hypothesis $H_0: \mu = \mu_0$, H_1 may by any one of the following three depending on the conjector of the researcher.

(i) $H_1: \mu \neq \mu_0$ or (ii) $H_1: \mu > \mu_0$ or (iii) $H_1: \mu < \mu_0$.

Test statistic is $Z_{cal} = \frac{(\bar{x} - \mu_0)}{\sigma/\sqrt{n}}$ is used to test H_0 against H_1.

Test Procedure or rule is based on Z which is standard normal. Taking α as level of significance, the critical regions are given by the following for the three alternatives;

a) If $H_1: \mu \neq \mu_0$, reject H_0 if $|Z_{CAL}| \geq Z_{\alpha/2}$.
b) If $H_1: \mu > \mu_0$, reject H_0 if $Z_{CAL} \geq Z_\alpha$.
c) If $H_1: \mu < \mu_0$, reject H_0 if $Z_{CAL} \leq -Z_\alpha$.

Example 3: Researcher is interested to answer the question whether the average enzyme level in a certain human population is different from 25. It is known that the said enzyme level (x) of interest is approximately normally distributed with variance of 45. The researcher selected sample of 10 individuals, determined enzyme level on each and calculated value of the sample mean which was 22. What should be the answer to the question of research on the basis of available sample observations?

Solution: Hypothesis to be tested is $H_0: \mu = 25$ against $H_1: \mu \neq 25$.

Given $n = 10$, $\bar{x} = 22$, $\sigma^2 = 45$.

Test statistic to be used is $Z_{CAL} = \dfrac{(\bar{x} - \mu_0)}{\sigma/\sqrt{n}} = \dfrac{22-25}{\sqrt{\dfrac{45}{10}}} = -1.41$.

Critical value is $Z_{\alpha/2} = 1.96$

Test procedure is if $|Z_{cal}| \geq Z_{\alpha/2}$, we reject H_0 at α % level of significance otherwise accept H_0.

Since $|Z_{cal}| = 1.41$ which is less than 1.96. Hence, we do not reject H_0 at 5% level of significance and conclude that the enzyme level in the studied population may not be different from 25.

Two sample problems for testing means: (large sample test i.e. n>30)
This section deals with problem of comparing means of a characteristic in two populations. From the two populations random samples of sizes n_1 and n_2 are selected and the value of the characteristic $\bar{x}_1$ and $\bar{x}_2$ are measured in the first and second populations respectively.

Assumptions:
The two populations are normally distributed with known variances σ^2_1 and σ^2_2 respectively and random samples of sizes n_1 and n_2 are selected independently from first and second populations respectively, with means μ_1 and μ_2 and known variances σ^2_1 and σ^2_2, n_1 and n_2 are large.
Test Procedures: Hypothesis $H_0: \mu_1 = \mu_2$, H_1 may be any one of the following three depending on the conjector of the researcher.
(i) $H_1: \mu_1 \neq \mu_2$ or (ii) $H_1: \mu_1 > \mu_2$ or (iii) $H_1: \mu_1 < \mu_2$.

Test statistics is $Z_{cal} = \dfrac{\bar{x}_1 - \bar{x}_2}{\sqrt{\dfrac{\sigma^2_1}{n_1} + \dfrac{\sigma^2_2}{n_2}}}$, where $\bar{x}_1$ and $\bar{x}_2$ are means of the first and second

samples respectively, is used to test H_0 against H_1.

Test procedure or rule is based on Z which is standard normal. Taking α as level of significance, the critical value are given by the following for the three alternatives;

a) If $H_1: \mu_1 \neq \mu_2$, reject H_0 if $|Z_{CAL}| \geq Z_{\alpha/2}$.
b) If $H_1: \mu_1 > \mu_2$, reject H_0 if $Z_{CAL} \geq Z_\alpha$.
c) If $H_1: \mu_1 < \mu_2$, reject H_0 if $Z_{CAL} \leq -Z_\alpha$.

Example 4: It is desired to know if the data provides evidence to indicate a difference in mean serum uric acid levels between normal individuals and individuals with mongolism. The uric acid level is known to follow normal distribution in both types of individual with variances 1. The random sample of 12 mongoloid and 15 normal individuals gave means as $\bar{x}_1 = 4.5$ mg/100 ml, $\bar{x}_2 = 3.4$ mg/100 ml.

Solution: Let x_1 and x_2 be the uric acid levels in the two groups of individuals. Given $n_1 = 12$ and $n_2 = 15$ and $\bar{x}_1 = 4.5$ mg/100 ml, $\bar{x}_2 = 3.4$ mg/100 ml, $\sigma_1^2 = 1$, $\sigma_2^2 = 1$.

Hypothesis to be tested is $H_0: \mu_1 = \mu_2$ against $H_1: \mu_1 \neq \mu_2$.

The test statistic to be used is

$$Z_{cal} = \frac{\bar{x}_1 - \bar{x}_2}{\sqrt{\frac{\sigma_1^2}{n_1} + \frac{\sigma_2^2}{n_2}}} = \frac{4.5 - 3.5}{\sqrt{\frac{1}{12} + \frac{1}{15}}} = 2.82.$$ Critical value is $Z_{\alpha/2} = 1.96$

Test procedure is if $|Z_{cal}| \geq Z_{\alpha/2}$, We reject H_0 at α % level of significance otherwise accept H_0.

Since $|Z_{cal}| = 2.82 \geq Z_{0.025} = 1.96$, hence, we reject H_0 at 5% level of significance and conclude that the data gives sufficient evidence to indicate that there is a significant difference in average serum uric acid levels in mongoloid and normal individuals at 5% level of significance.

Small sample tests (Exact sampling distributions):

If the sample size n is small (n<30) the sampling distribution of statistics cannot be approximated by standard normal distribution. In such cases exact sample tests, pioneered by W.S. Gosset (1908) who wrote under the pen name of the student, and later on developed and extended by prof. R. A. Fisher (1926) are used.

Few test based on small sample tests are as follows:

1. Student's t–distribution.
2. Chi-square (x^2) distribution.
3. Snedecor's F-distribution.

The exact sample tests can, however, be applied to large samples also though the converse is not true. In all the exact sample tests, the basic assumption is that "the population(s) from which sample(s) is (are) drawn is(are) normal."

Student's t–distribution:

Student's t–distribution is a continuous probability distribution, used for testing of hypothesis for small sample size (n<30).

Let $x_1, x_2, \ldots, x_n$ be a random sample of size n from a normal population with mean μ and variance σ^2 then student's t variable is defined by

$$t_{cal} = \frac{\overline{x} - \mu}{\frac{s}{\sqrt{n}}}, \text{ where } \overline{x} = \frac{\sum\limits_{i=1}^{n} x_i}{n}, \text{ is the sample mean and } S^2 = \frac{\sum\limits_{i=1}^{n} (x_i - \overline{x})^2}{n-1} \text{ is an}$$

unbiased estimate of the population variance σ^2, and it follows student's t-distribution with (n-1) degrees of freedom.

Note: The student's t–distribution is symmetric, more peaked than normal distribution for large degrees of freedom of t tends to normal distribution.

Applications of Student's t–distribution:

1. Test for specified mean.
2. Test for comparison of mean of two independent samples.
3. Paired t-test for differences of means.

t-test for specified mean :

Let $x_1, x_2, \ldots, x_n$ be a random sample drawn from a normal distribution with population mean μ and unknown variance σ^2 to test whether the population mean is equal to specific mean μ_0. Test procedures: Hypothesis $H_0: \mu = \mu_0$, H_1 may by any one of the following three depending on the conjector of the researcher.

(i) $H_1: \mu \neq \mu_0$ or (ii) $H_1: \mu > \mu_0$ or (iii) $H_1: \mu < \mu_0$.

Test statistic is $t_{cal} = \frac{\overline{x} - \mu_0}{\frac{s}{\sqrt{n}}}$ is used to test H_0 against H_1, where $\overline{x} = \frac{\sum\limits_{i=1}^{n} x_i}{n}$, and

$s^2 = \frac{\sum_{i=1}^{n}(x_i - \overline{x})^2}{n-1}$, follows student's t-distribution with n-1 degrees of freedom.

Test Procedure or rule is based on student's t-distribution. Taking α as level of significance, the critical values are given by the following for the three alternatives;

a) If $H_1 : \mu \neq \mu_0$, reject H_0 if $|t_{cal}| \geq t_{n-1,\alpha/2}$.

b) If $H_1 : \mu > \mu_0$, reject H_0 if $t_{cal} \geq t_{n-1,\alpha}$.

c) If $H_1 : \mu < \mu_0$, reject H_0 if $t_{cal} \leq -t_{n-1,\alpha}$.

We use above test to test hypothesis as

i)   The target weight of a batch of tablets is 325 mg (specification weight).

ii)   An antihypertensive agent is hypothesized to lower the blood pressure by 10 mm Hg. on an average.

iii) The specification for disintegration time of tablets is not more than 15 min ($H_0 : \mu \leq 15$ min)

Example 5: Tablet weights (mg) of 20 randomly selected tablets are as follows :

300, 320, 306, 310, 316, 317, 316, 319, 320, 325, 325, 321, 321, 322, 323, 325, 327, 331, 336, 320. Test the hypothesis that mean weight of tablets is 325 mg at 5% level of significance?

Solution: Given n=20, hypothesis to be test is $H_0 : \mu = 325$ mg and $H_1 : \mu \neq 325$ mg.

From above data, $\bar{x} = \dfrac{\sum\limits_{i=1}^{n} x_i}{n} = \dfrac{(300+320+\ldots\ldots+320)}{2} = 319.75$ mg and

$S^2 = \dfrac{\sum\limits_{i=1}^{n} (x_i - \bar{x})^2}{n-1}$ 67.2 and $S = \sqrt{S^2} = 8.197560$.

Test statistics to be used is

$$t_{cal} = \dfrac{\bar{x} - \mu_0}{\dfrac{S}{\sqrt{n}}} \sim t_{n-1}$$

$$= \dfrac{319.75 - 325}{8.197560/\sqrt{20}} = 2.86411 .$$

Test procedure is reject H_0 at 5% level of significance if $|t_{cal}| \geq t_{n-1,\,\alpha/2}$, otherwise accept H_0.

Here, $|t_{cal}| = 2.86411 > t_{19,0.025} = 2.09$, hence we reject H_0 at 5% level of significance and conclude that the average batch weight of 20 tablets is approximately 319.75

mg which is sufficiently far from the target weight of 325 mg weight to declare a significant difference.

t-test to compare means of two independent samples:

Let $x_1, x_2, \ldots, x_n$ be a random sample of size $n_1 (<30)$ drawn from a normal population with unknown mean μ_1 and unknown variance σ_1^2. Let $y_1, y_2, \ldots, y_n$ be a random sample of size $n_2 (<30)$ drawn independently from another normal population with unknown mean μ_2 and unknown variance σ_2^2 assuming $\sigma^2 = \sigma_1^2 = \sigma_2^2$.

Test procedure is Hypothesis $H_0: \mu_1 = \mu_2$, H_1 may be any one of the following three depending on the conjector of the researcher.

(i) $H_1: \mu_1 \neq \mu_2$ or (ii) $H_1: \mu_1 > \mu_2$ or (iii) $H_1: \mu_1 < \mu_2$.

Test statistics is $t_{cal} = \dfrac{\bar{x} - \bar{y}}{S * \sqrt{\dfrac{1}{n_1} + \dfrac{1}{n_2}}}$, is used to test H_0 against H_1, where $\bar{x} = \dfrac{\sum\limits_{i=1}^{n} x_i}{n}$, $\bar{y} = \dfrac{\sum\limits_{i=1}^{n} y_i}{n}$

$S^2 = \dfrac{n_1 S_1^2 + n_2 S_2^2}{n_1 + n_2 - 2}$, and $S_1^{\,2} = \dfrac{\sum\limits_{i=1}^{n} (x_i - \bar{x})^2}{n_1}$, $S_2^{\,2} = \dfrac{\sum\limits_{j=1}^{n} (y_j - \bar{y})^2}{n_2}$,

Test procedure or rule is based on student's t-distributions with $(n_1 + n_2 - 2)$ degrees of freedom. Taking α as level of significance, the critical value are given by the following for the three alternatives;

a) If $H_1: \mu \neq \mu_0$, reject H_0 if $|t_{cal}| \geq t_{n_1 + n_2 - 2, \alpha/2}$.

b) If $H_1: \mu > \mu_0$, reject H_0 if $t_{cal} \geq t_{n_1 + n_2 - 2, \alpha}$.

c) If $H_1: \mu < \mu_0$, reject H_0 if $t_{cal} \leq -t_{n_1 + n_2 - 2, \alpha}$.

Example 6: A study of angina, on rats was conducted on 18 rats with a history of angina. These 18 rats were split randomly into two groups of 9 each. One group was given a placebo (control) and the other an experimental drug FL. After controlled exercise on a tread mill, the recovery time of each rat was determined. The following information is available:

	Sample size	Mean	Sample variance
Control	9	329 seconds	45 seconds
FL	9	283 seconds	43 seconds

Do the data support the convention that FL 113 will reduce the average recovery time? Recovery time may assumed to be normal.

Solution: Given n1=9, n2=9, $\bar{x}=329$, $\bar{y}=283$ and $S_1^2 = 45$ and $S_2^2 = 43$, hypothesis to be used is $H_0: \mu_1 = \mu_2$ against $H_1: \mu_1 > \mu_2$.

Test statistic to be used is

$$t_{cal} = \frac{\bar{x}-\bar{y}}{s* \sqrt{\frac{1}{n_1}+\frac{1}{n_2}}} = \frac{329-283}{\sqrt{44\frac{1}{9}+\frac{1}{9}}} = 14.71 \text{ and } S^2 = \frac{n_1 S_1^2 + n_2 S_2^2}{n_1+n_2-2} = \frac{8(45)+8(43)}{9+9-2} = 44.$$

Test procedure is reject H_0 if $t_{cal} \geq t_{16,0.05} = 1.746$.

Since $t_{cal} \geq t_{16,0.05} = 1.746$, therefore reject H_0 at 5% level of significance.

Hence it can be concluded that the drug FL 113 is effective in reducing recovery time.

Remark: Thus before applying t-test for testing the equality of means it is therotically desirable to the test the equality of population variances by applying F-test. If the variances do not come out to be equal the t-test becomes invalid and in that case Behren's 'd'-test based on confidence interval is used. For practical problems, however, the assumptions of normality and equality of variances of two populations are taken for granted.

Paired t-test:

When we deal with data of the type before and after or paired data then the two samples are not independent. In this case, we work with signed differences of paired data and test whether these differences may be looked as a random sample from a normal distribution for which mean is zero.

If the paired sample is of small size i.e. n<30 we use one sample t-test concerning mean and call it as paired t-test.

Examples of paired to test are:

To study the effect of physical training of the serum cholesterol level, on 11 subjects before and after the training program.

Let (x_i, y_i) i=1,2,...n be pair of observations recorded on n ($\leq$30) individuals at two different times. (x_i, y_i) follow normal distribution with means μ_1 and μ_2 and variances σ_1^2 and σ_2^2 respectively.

Here, we consider the differences between x_i and y_i, $d_i = x_i - y_i$, $i = 1,2,\ldots.n$. Under the null hypothesis H_0 that population mean differences is not significant.
Test statistics to test H_0 is given by

$$t_{cal} = \frac{\bar{d}}{\frac{S_d}{\sqrt{n}}}, \text{ Where } \bar{d} = \frac{\sum_{i=1}^{n} d_i}{n} \text{ and } S_d^2 = \frac{\sum_{i=1}^{n} (d_i - \bar{d})^2}{n-1}.$$

Under the null hypothesis H_0, the distribution of the test stantistics follows t-distribution with $(n-1)$ degrees of freedom, if H_0 is true.

Test procedure or rule is given by
a) Reject H_0 if $H_1 : \mu_1 \neq \mu_2$, reject H_0 if $|t_{cal}| \geq t_{n-1,\alpha/2}$.
b) Reject H_0 if $H_1 : \mu_1 > \mu_2$, reject H_0 if $t_{cal} \geq t_{n-1,\alpha}$.
c) Reject H_0 if $H_1 : \mu_1 < \mu_2$, reject H_0 if $t_{cal} \leq -t_{n-1,\alpha}$.

Example 7: On hot plate analgesiometer Tail flick latency was measured before and after administration of narcotic analgesic, Morphine.

Serial Number	Tail flick Latency (seconds) before administration of Morphine	Tail flick Latency (seconds) after administration of Morphine
1	3	10
2	4	12
3	2	9
4	4	11
5	2	8
6	3	9
Mean	**3.16**	**11.33**

Test whether is there any of change in tail flick latency after the administration of narcotic analgesic Morphine.

Solution: We require to test the effect of administration of narcotic analgesic morphine. Hence we use paired t test. H_0: There is significant difference between tail flick latency (seconds) after administration of morphine.

Against H_1: There is no significant difference between tail flick latency (seconds) after administration of morphine.

Serial Number	Tail flick Latency (seconds) before administration of Morphine x_i	Tail flick Latency (seconds) after administration of Morphine y_i	$d = x_i - y_i$	d^2
1	3	10	-7	49
2	4	12	-8	64
3	2	9	-7	49
4	4	11	-7	49
5	2	8	-6	36
6	3	9	-6	36
Total			$\sum d_i = -41$	$\sum d_i^2 = 283$

$$\overline{d} = \frac{\sum d_i}{n} = \frac{-41}{6} = 6.8333 \text{ and}$$

$$S_d^2 = \frac{\sum_{i=1}^{n} (d_i - \overline{d})^2}{n-1} = \frac{18038.67653}{5} = 3607.735307, S_d = 60.0644263 \cdot$$

Test statistics is

$$t_{cal} = \frac{\overline{d}}{\frac{S_d}{\sqrt{n}}} = \frac{-6.833}{\frac{60.0644263}{\sqrt{6}}} = \frac{-6.833}{24.52119935} = -0.278669077 \quad.$$

Critical value for $t_{n-1,\alpha/2} = t_{5,.025} = 2.571$.

Test procedure is to reject H_0 at 5% level of significance if $|t_{cal}| \geq t_{n-1,\alpha/2}$, otherwise accept H_0.

Since $|t_{cal}| = 0.278669077$ which is less than $t_{n-1,\alpha/2} = t_{5,.025} = 2.571$, therefore, do not reject H_0 at 5% level of significance.

There is significance difference between tail flick latency (seconds) after administration of morphine.

Chi-square distribution (x^2):

Let $x_1, x_2, \ldots, x_n$ be independent normal variables and $X_i \sim N(\mu_i, \sigma_i^2)$ $i = 1, 2, \ldots, n$ then

$$x^2 = \sum_{i=1}^{n} \left(\frac{x_i - \mu_i}{\sigma_i}\right)^2 \text{ is a chi-square}$$

Variable with n degrees of freedom thus x^2 variable is defined as sum of squares of standard normal variable. It is a continuous probability distribution. Chi-square distribution is positively skewed distribution. Its application is for testing independence of attributes.

Chi-square test for independence of attributes

Chi-square test for independence of attributes is used to test independence of two attributes. Let the data be classified into 'm' classes $A_1, A_2, \ldots, A_n$ according to attribute A and into 'n' classes according to attribute B thus we have (m×n) contingency table as below:

B ╲ A	$B_1, B_2, \ldots, B_j, \ldots B_n$	Total
A_1	$O_{11}, O_{12}, \ldots, O_{1j}, \ldots O_{1n}$	R_1
A_2	$O_{21}, O_{22}, \ldots, O_{2j}, \ldots, O_{2n}$	R_2
⋮		⋮
⋮		⋮
A_i	$O_{i1}, O_{i2}, \ldots, O_{ij}, \ldots, O_{in}$	R_i
⋮		⋮
⋮		⋮
A_m	$O_{m1}, O_{m2}, \ldots, O_{mj}, \ldots, O_{mn}$	R_m
Total	$C_1 \quad C_2 \quad C_j C_n$	$N = \sum_{i=1}^{2} R_i = \sum_{j=1}^{2} C_j$

O_{ij} : Observed frequency of the cell belong to i^{th} row of A and j^{th} column of B.

Let R_i : Total of frequencies in i^{th} row.

C_j: Total of frequencies in j^{th} column.

Test procedure is to test H_0: Attributes A and B are independent against H_1: Attributes A and B are not independent.

Let α be level of significance.

Expected frequencies of $(i,j)^{th}$ cell is given by

$$E_{ij} = \frac{(R_i) \times (C_j)}{N}; i=1,2,..,m; j=1,2,...,n$$

Test statistics to be used is

$$\chi^2_{cal} = \sum_{i=1}^{m} \sum_{j=1}^{n} \left(\frac{(o_{ij}-E_{ij})^2}{E_{ij}} \right) = \sum_{i=1}^{m} \sum_{j=1}^{n} \frac{o_{ij}^2}{E_{ij}} - N,$$

and it follows chi-square distribution with $(m-1) \times (n-1)$ degrees of freedom.

Test procedure is to reject H_0 at α % level of significance if $\chi^2_{cal} \geq \chi^2_{(m-1)(n-1),\alpha}$, otherwise accept H_0.

Example 8: Consider following preclinical study performed to determine the carcinogenic potency of a new drug in which 100 control animals were compared to a group of 100 animals given the drug. At the end of experiment, the animals were examined for tumors. Ten animals in the control group and eight in the drug treated group, died of non drug related courses and these animals were not included in the final count. Test whether there is an association between drug given to animal.

	Numbers with tumors	Number without tumors	Total
Drug	18	74	92
Placebo	14	76	90
Total	32	150	182

Solution: Test procedure is to test H_0 : There is no association between drug given to animal and animal developed tumor against H_1: There is association between drug given to animal and animal developed tumor.

Let α be 5% level of significance.

Table of observed frequency are given below:

	Numbers with tumors	Number without tumors	Total
Drug	18	74	92
Placebo	14	76	90
Total	32	150	182

Expected frequency is given by $E_{ij} = \frac{R_i \times C_j}{N}$, Ri : i^{th} row total; i=1,2, C_j: j^{th} column total; j=1,2 and $N = \sum_{i=1}^{2} R_i = \sum_{j=1}^{2} C_j$.

Thus table of expected frequency is:

	Numbers with tumors	Number without tumors	Total
Drug	16.18	75.82	92
Placebo	15.82	74.18	90
Total	32	150	182

Test statistics to be used is

$$x^2_{cal} = \sum_{i=1}^{2} \sum_{j=1}^{2} \left(\frac{(o_{ij} - E_{ij})^2}{E_{ij}} \right) = \frac{(18-16.18)^2}{16.18} + \frac{(74-75.82)^2}{75.82} + \frac{(14-15.82)^2}{15.82} + \frac{(76-74.18)^2}{74.18} = 0.50244.$$

Under H_0,

test statistics x^2_{cal} has chi-square distribution with $(2-1)(2-1)=1$ degrees of freedom.
Critical value $= x^2_{(2-1)(2-1),0.05} = x^2_{1,0.05} = 3.84$.

Test procedure is to reject H_0 if $x^2_{cal} \geq x^2_{1.0.05} = 3.84$, otherwise accept H_0.
Since from the above data $x^2_{cal} < x^2_{1.0.05} = 3.84$, therefore we do not reject H_0.

Thus there is association between drug given to animals and tumors caused by animals at 5% level of significance.

Snedecor's F distribution:

Definition:

Let X and Y be two independent chi-square variable with n_1 and n_2 degrees of freedom respectively, then F-statistic is F with (n_1, n_2) degrees of freedom is defined as

$$F = \frac{X/n_1}{Y/n_2}$$

In other words, F is defined as the ration of two independent chi-square variables divided by theie respective degrees of freedom and it follows Snedecor's F distribution with (n_1, n_2) degrees of freedom. F distribution is highly positively skewed distribution.

Applications of F-distributions:

F-test for equality of variances of two populations:
Let $x_1, x_2, \ldots, x_n$ be a random sample of n_1 $(n_1 < 30)$ drawn from a normal population with unknown variance σ_1^2. Let $y_1, y_2, \ldots, y_n$ be a random sample of n_2 $(n_2 < 30)$ drawn from another normal distribution with unknown variance σ_2^2.

Hypothesis to be tested is $H_0: \sigma_1^2 = \sigma_2^2$ against one of the following three alternatives as (i) $H_1: \sigma_1^2 \neq \sigma_2^2$ or (ii) $H_1: \sigma_1^2 > \sigma_2^2$ or (iii) $H_1: \sigma_1^2 < \sigma_2^2$.

The test statistics for testing H_0 is

$$F_{cal} = \frac{S_1^2}{S_2^2} \text{ if } S_1^2 > S_2^2$$

$$= \frac{S_2^2}{S_1^2} \text{ if } S_2^2 > S_1^2,$$

Where $S_1^2 = \dfrac{\sum\limits_{i=1}^{n_1} (x_i - \bar{x})^2}{n_1 - 1}$, $S_2^2 = \dfrac{\sum\limits_{j=1}^{n_2} (y_j - \bar{y})^2}{n_2 - 1}$, and it follows F-distribution with (n_1, n_2)

degrees of freedom, if H_0 is true.

The test procedure or rule depends on the following alternatives as

(i) Reject H_0 if $F_{cal} \geq F_{n_1-1, n_2-1, \alpha/2}$ if $H_1: \sigma_1^2 \neq \sigma_2^2$.

(ii) Reject H_0 if $F_{cal} \geq F_{n_1-1, n_2-1, \alpha}$ if $H_1: \sigma_1^2 > \sigma_2^2$.

(iii) Reject H_0 if $F_{cal} \geq F_{n_1-1, n_2-1, 1-\alpha}$ if $H_1: \sigma_1^2 < \sigma_2^2$.

Example 9: Heart rate is measured in Sprague Dawley male and female rats.

Heart rate in beats per minute	
Male wistar rats	**Female wistar rats**
323	377
330	385
345	367
335	392
315	415
355	430

Test whether two samples taken from random population have the same variance at 5% level of significance.

Solution: Test procedure is to test H_0: there is no significant difference between variances of two population against H_1: there is a significant difference between variances of two population.

Given that $\alpha = 0.05$, from the above data, for male wistar rats, we have

$$\bar{x} = \frac{\sum_1^6 x_i}{6} = \frac{2003}{6} = 333.8333 \text{ and for female wistar rats we have}$$

$$\bar{y} = \frac{\sum_1^6 y_j}{6} = \frac{2366}{6} = 394.3333 \quad , \quad S_1^2 = \frac{\sum\limits_{i=1}^{n_1} (x_i - \bar{x})^2}{n_1 - 1} = \frac{1060.826833}{5} = 212.1653667$$

and $$S_2^2 = \frac{\sum\limits_{j=1}^{n_2} (y_j - \bar{y})^2}{n_2 - 1} = \frac{2839.311934}{5} = 567.8623868 \quad \cdot$$

Since $s_1^2 < s_2^2$.

The test statistics is

$$F_{cal} = \frac{S_2^2}{S_1^2} \text{ if } S_2^2 > S_1^2$$

$$= \frac{567.8623868}{212.1653667} = 2.676508403 \quad .$$

Critical value is $F_{5,5,0.05} = 5.05$.

Test procedure is if $F_{cal} \geq F_{n_1-1,n_2-1,\alpha/2}$ then reject H_0 at $\alpha\%$ level of significance, otherwise accept H_0.

Since $F_{cal} = 2.676508403 < F_{5,5,0.05} = 5.05$.

Hence we do not reject H_0 at 5% level of significance.

$\therefore$ There is no significant difference between variances of two population of male wistar rats and female wistar rats.

Analysis of variance (ANOVA)

ANOVA deals with comparison among given number of effects within themselves. The one-way analysis of variance (ANOVA) is used to determine whether there are any statistically significant differences between the means of two or more independent (unrelated) groups. It is used specifically to test the homogenity between two groups or more than two groups depending on the situations. For example, you could use a one-way ANOVA to understand difference in exam performance among students by using test on anxiety levels during which students can be divided into three independent groups (e.g., low, medium and high-stressed students). Also, it is important to realize that the one-way ANOVA is an **omnibus** test statistic and cannot tell you which specific groups were statistically significantly different from each other; it only tells you that at least two groups were different. Since you may have three, four, five or more groups in your study design, determining which of these groups differ from each other is important.

There are some assumptions in analysis of variance technique.

1. Normality i.e the values in each group(part) are normally distributed.
2. Homogeneity i.e. the variance within each group should be equal for all groups. This assumption is needed in order to contribute or pool the variances within the groups into a single "within groups" source of variation.
3. Independence of error: It states that the error (variation of each value and its own group mean) should be independent for each value.

In one way ANOVA the data are classified according to only one criterion. We are considering influence only one factor.

Under the null hypothesis we have
$\alpha_1 = \alpha_2 = \ldots\ldots = \alpha_k = 0$

let us assume that N observation xij (i=1,2,….k), j=(1,2,..n_j) of a random variable X are grouped according to some criterion into k classes of sizes $n_1, n_2, \ldots., n_k$ respectively.

Classes	1	2	3	…..	K	Total
Observations	X_{11}	X_{21}	X_{31}		X_{k1}	
	X_{12}	X_{22}	X_{32}		X_{K2}	
	X_{13}	X_{23}	X_{33}		X_{K3}	
	:	:	:		:	
	:	:	:		:	
	X_{1j}	X_{2j}	X_{3j}		X_{Kj}	
	:	:	:		:	
	:	:	:		:	
Total	T_1	T_2	T_3		T_K	GRAND TOTAL=T
Means	$\bar{x}_1$	$\bar{x}_2$	$\bar{x}_3$		$\bar{x}_K$	

In one way analysis of variance
To test H_0: there is no significance difference between class means.
Against H_1 : there is significance difference between class means.
i.e. to test H_0: $\mu_1 = \mu_2 = \ldots = \mu_k$ against $H_1 : \mu_1 \neq \mu_2 \neq \ldots \neq \mu_k$
here we assume that x_{ij} is assumed to be made of different components.

$X_{ij} = \mu + \alpha_i + \epsilon_{ij}$; i=1,2,...k, j=1,2,...n_j. Where μ = overall mean or general mean α_i = effect of ith group population, ϵ_{ij} = error term

In one–way analysis of variance we require to calculate the following terms.

Calculate=correction factor=C.F=$\frac{T^2}{N}$ where T: grand total, N = total number of observations.

Calculate sum of squares between classes = sum of squares between columns $= \sum_{i=1}^{k} (\bar{x}_i - \bar{\bar{x}})^2$, where $\bar{x}_i$ = mean of ith sample and grand average = N, n_i :i^{th} class size.

Sum of squares between classes=sum of squares between column =

CSS $= \frac{C_1^2}{n_1} + \frac{C_2^2}{n_2} + \cdots\cdots + \frac{C_k^2}{n_k}$ -C.F

Total sum of squares=TSS=sum of squares of each observation-

C.F= $\sum_{i=1}^{k} \sum_{j=1}^{ni} (x_{ij})^2 - \frac{T^2}{N}$

Sum of squares of variation within or error sum of square=ESS=TSS-CSS

	Sum of Squares	d.f.	Mean Square	F ratio
Between classes (CSS)	CSS	k-1	MSC= $\frac{CSS}{k-1}$	MSC/MSE
Error	ESS	N-k	MSE= $\frac{ESS}{N-K}$	
Total	TSS	N-1		

Critical value for above test is $F_{(k-1),\,(n-k),\alpha}$ such that if F ratio $\geq F_{(k-1),\,(n-k),\alpha}$ we reject H_0 at α % level of significance, otherwise accept it.

Example 10: In a preclinical study, 18 animals were randomly divided into three groups, each group containing six animals. Group 1 was control which was treated with vehicle alone whereas group 2 and 3 were treated with two antihypertensive experimental drugs 1 and 2 respectively. One animal died from the Control group. The results (change in blood pressure from baseline) are shown in following table. (Use 5% level of significance).

Control	Drug 1	Drug 2
14	15	8
16	12	14
20	19	13
22	11	6
16	12	14
20	15	8

Do the observed differences merely reflect the inherent variation of the animals response to such treatment? Use 5% level of significance.

Solution: Test procedure is to test H_0: there are no observed differences in treatment means and Against H_1: there is observed differences in treatment means.
Table:

Control	Drug 1	Drug 2	
14	15	8	
16	12	14	
20	19	13	
22	11	6	
16	12	14	
20	15	8	
108	84	63	Grand total = 255

Correction factor = C.F. = $\dfrac{T^2}{N}$, where T = grand total, N = total number of observations,

C.F. = $\dfrac{T^2}{N} = \dfrac{(255)^2}{18} = 3612.5$

Sum of squares between columns

$= \dfrac{C_1^2}{n_1} + \dfrac{C_2^2}{n_2} + \dfrac{C_3^2}{n_3}$ - C.F = $\dfrac{108^2}{6} + \dfrac{84^2}{6} + \dfrac{63^2}{6} - 3612.5 = 169 = $ CSS.

Total sum of squares = sum of squares of each observation -

C.F. = 3937 - 3612.5 = 324.5 = TSS.

SSE = TSS - CSS = 155.5.

ANOVA table

Source of variation	Degrees of freedom	Sum of squares	Mean sum of squares	F ratio
Between columns /groups	2=(3-1)	169	$\dfrac{169}{2}=84.5$	$\dfrac{84.5}{10.3666}=8.1511$
Error	17-2=15	155.5	$\dfrac{155.5}{15}=10.3666$	
Total	18-1=17	324.5		

Test procedure to be used is if F ratio $\geq F_{2,8,0.5}$ (table value), we reject H_0 at 5% level of significance, otherwise accept H_0.

Here $F_{2,15,0.05}$ = 4.46 (F table value), since 8.1511 > $F_{2,8,0.5}$ = 4.46, therefore, reject H_0 at 5% level of significance.

Therefore, the treatment means differs from each other at 5% level of significance.

Two way Analysis of Variance (ANOVA)

The two-way analysis of variance is an extension to the one-way analysis of variance. There are two independent variables (hence the name two-way). There are, however, many situations in which the response variable of interest may be affected by more than one factor. For example, sales of max factor cosmetics may be affected by the point-of-scale, the price charged, the size and/or location of store or the number of competitive products. Thus it is possible to design the test so that analysis of variance can be used to test for the effects of two factors simultaneously such a test is called two-factor analysis of variance or two–way analysis of variance.

Assumptions

* The populations from which the samples were obtained must be normally or approximately normally distributed.
* The samples must be independent.
* The variances of the populations must be equal.
* The groups must have the same sample size.

The N observation is divided into rows according to one factor and columns according to other factor. In two way analysis, total sum of squares is split into three parts:

1. Sum of squares between column = CSS.
2. Sum of squares within rows = RSS.
3. Sum of squares due to error = SSE.

Observations are grouped as:

Factor 2 / Factor 1	1	2	3	.....	C	Total	Means
Observations	X_{11}	X_{21}	X_{31}		X_{c1}	R_1	$\bar{x}_1$
	X_{12}	X_{22}	X_{32}		X_{c2}	R_2	$\bar{x}_2$
	X_{13}	X_{23}	X_{33}		X_{c3}	R_3	$\bar{x}_3$
	:	:	:		:		
	:	:	:		:		
	X_{1j}	X_{2j}	X_{3j}		X_{cj}	R_j	$\bar{x}_l$
	:	:	:		:		
	$:X_{r1}$	$:X_{r2}$	$:X_{r3}$		$:X_{rc}$	R_r	$\bar{x}_r$
Total	C_1	C_2	C_3		C_c	**GRAND TOTAL=T**	
Means	$\bar{x}_{.1}$	$\bar{x}_{.2}$	$\bar{x}_{.3}$		$\bar{x}_{.c}$		

To test: H_{01}: there is no significant difference between means of factor 2 (between column). H_{02}: there is no significant difference between means of factor 1 (between rows) in two way classification the analysis of variance table takes the following terms:

Source	SS	d.f	MS	F
Between Columns	CSS	c-1	CSS / (c-1) =MSC	MSC / MSE
Within rows	RSS	r-1	RSS / (r-1) = MSR	MSR / MSE
Error	$SSE=TSS-CSS-RSS$	(r-1)(c-1)	MSE / (r-1) (c-1) =MSE	
Total	TSS	rc - 1,		

where, correction factor $= C.F = \dfrac{T^2}{N}$, T = Grand total, N = total number of observations, c = number of columns, r = number of rows.

$$SSC = \frac{C_1^2}{n_1} + \frac{C_2^2}{n_2} + \cdots\cdots + \frac{C_c^2}{n_c} - C.F \text{ and } SSR = \frac{R_1^2}{n_1} + \frac{R_2^2}{n_2} + \frac{R_3^2}{n_3} + \frac{R_4^2}{n_4} + \cdots\cdots + \frac{R_r^2}{n_r} - C.F$$

Where R_i: row total for factor 1, Cj: column total for factor 2, n_i: no. of elements in i^{th} row of factor 1, n_j : no. of elements of jth column of factor 2

TSS = sum of square of each observations - C.F.

SSE = TSS - (SSC+SSR).

Critical value: for H_{01} is $F_{(c-1),(r-1)(c-1),\alpha}$

Such that if F ratio for columns is $\geq F_{(c-1),(r-1)(c-1),\alpha}$

We reject H_{01}

For H_{02} is $F_{(r-1),(r-1)(c-1),\alpha}$

Such that if F ratio for rows is $\geq F_{(r-1),(r-1)(c-1),\alpha}$

We reject H_{02}, at α % level of significance.

Example 11: The data given below are plasma calcium concentration (in mg/100ml) of birds of both sexes. The birds of each sex are being treated with hormone. Perform ANOVA and test the hypothesis that the average plasma calcium concentration of birds in the sampled population is not affected by hormone treatment and sex of the bird.

Hormone treatment	Female	Male
1	39.1	32.0
2	26.2	23.8
3	21.3	28.8
4	35.8	25.0
5	40.2	29.3

Solution:

H_0: There is no effect of hormone treatment on mean plasma calcium concentration
Against

H_{02}: male and female (i.e. sex of) birds have no difference in mean plasma calcium concentration.

Hormone treatment	Female	Male	Total
1	39.1	32.0	71.1
2	26.2	23.8	50
3	21.3	28.8	50.1
4	35.8	25	60.8
5	40.2	29.3	69.5
Total	162.6	138.9	T=grand total=301.5

$N=10$ correction factor = C.F = $\frac{T^2}{N} = \frac{(301.5)^2}{10} = 9090.225$.

Between male and female SS = SSC = $\frac{C_1^2}{n_1} + \frac{C_2^2}{n_2}$ - C.F

$$= \frac{162.6^2}{5} + \frac{138.9^2}{5} - 9090.225 = 56.169 = CSS.$$

Between batches s = SSR = $\frac{R_1^2}{n_1} + \frac{R_2^2}{n_2} + \frac{R_3^2}{n_3} + \frac{R_4^2}{n_4} + \frac{R_5^2}{n_5}$ - C.F

$$= \frac{71.1^2}{2} + \frac{50^2}{2} + \frac{50.1^2}{2} + \frac{60.8^2}{2} + \frac{69.5^2}{2} - 9090.225 = 205.83 = RSS.$$

TSS = sum of squares of each observation - C.F. = 9469.99 - 9090.225 = 379.765.

Errors SS = SSE = TSS - SSC - SSR = 117.766.

ANOVA TABLE

S.V	d.f	S.S	MSS	F ratio
SSR	5-1=4	205.83	51.4575	1.747
SSc	2-1=1	56.169	56.169	0.4769
Error SS	4	117.766	29.4415	
Total SS	10-1=9	379.765		

Test statistic to be used is Decision for H_{01} : $F_1 = 1.47$ which is less than $F_{4,4,0.05}$ =6.39. Hence we do not reject H_{01} at 5% level of significance.

There is no effect of hormone treatment on mean plasma calcium concentration.

Decision for H_{02} : $F_2 = 0.4769$ which is less than $F_{1,4,0.05} = 7.71$. Hence do not reject H_{02} at 5% level of significance.

$\therefore$ Male and Female (i.e. sex of) birds have no difference in mean plasma calcium concentration.

Tukey test:

The Tukey test (or Tukey procedure), also called Tukey honest significant difference test, is a post-hoc test based on studentized range distribution. An ANOVA test can tell you if your results are significant overall, but won't tell you exactly where those differences lie. Tukey test is used to find out which specific group's means (compared with each other) are different. The test compares all possible pairs of means.

Assumptions:

1. Observations are independent within and among groups.
2. The groups for each mean in the test are normally distributed.
3. There is equal within-group variance across the groups associated with each mean in the test (homogeneity of variance).

Method:

Calculate $\text{HSD} = \dfrac{M_i - M_j}{\sqrt{\dfrac{MS_W}{nh}}}$

Where $M_i - M_j$ is the difference between the pair of means. To calculate this, M_i should be larger than M_j.

MS_w is the mean square within, and n is the number in the group or treatment.

Step 1: Perform the ANOVA test. Assuming your F value is significant. You can run the post hoc test.

Step 2: Choose two means from the ANOVA output.

Note the following:

1. Means, 2. Means square within, 3. Number per treatment /group, 4. Degrees of freedom.

Step 3: Calculate the HSD statistic for the Tukey test using the formula.

Step 4: Find the score in Tukey's critical value table.

Step 5: Compare the score you calculated in step 3 with the tabulated value you found in.

Step 6: If the calculated value from step 3 is bigger than the critical value from the critical value table, the two means are significantly different.

Dunnett test:

Dunnett test is one of a number of a posteriori or post hoc tests, run after a significant one-way analysis of variance (ANOVA), to determine which differences are significant. The procedure was introduced by Charles W. Dunnett in 1955. It differs from other post hoc tests, such as the Newman–Keuls test, Duncan's Multiple Range test, Scheffé's test, or Tukey's Honestly Significant Difference test, because its use is restricted to compare a number of experimental groups against a single control group; it does not test the experimental groups against one another. Background information, the process of running Dunnett test, and an example are provided in this entry. Dunnett test (also called Dunnett method or Dunnett multiple comparisons) compares means from several experimental groups against a control group mean to find out the difference in these groups. When an ANOVA test has significant findings, it doesn't report which pairs are different. Dunnett can be used after the ANOVA has been run to identify the pairs with significant differences.

One fixed "control" group is compared to all the other samples, so it should be used when you have a control group. If you don't have a control group, use Tukey test.

As Dunnett compares two groups, it acts similarly to a t-test. The following formula gives value that can be used to compare mean differences. The formula is:

$$D_{dunnett} = t_{dunnett} \sqrt{\frac{2\,MS_{S/A}}{n}}$$

Step 1: Look up the $t_{dunnett}$ critical value in the dunnett-crtical value table. Choose your $\alpha = 0.05$, sample size n, degrees of freedom from the ANOVA "within groups" output. Plug the value in the formula of D.

Step 2: Find the mean squares within group in the ANOVA source table. Plug that value into the above formula.

Step 3: Find 'n' in one group. For this, If the difference between a control group mean and an experimental group mean is greater than $D_{dunnett}$ value then that difference is significant.

Non Parametric Test:

Parameter: It is a summary value or numerical index like mean,median, standard deviations or variance of a variable for the entire population.

Parametric test: Most commonly used statistical methods are called parametric because they are involved in testing the values of parameter (mean median or standard deviation). In parametric test it is assumed that population is normally distributed. Tests which are discussed earlier are parametric tests.

Non-Parametric test: Non –parametric test or methods are mathematical procedures concerned with the treatment of standard statistical problems when the assumptions of normality is not valid by general assumption concerning the distribution function. It is also called distribution free test. In addition analysis of data using non-parametric methods has the advantage of using simple calculation that are often based on ordering or ranking procedures. Thus, these methods can be used to obtain a quick look before a full-fledged analysis is undertaken. The disadvantages is that these tests lack power compared with corresponding parametric tests and these tests are not preferred when sample size gets larger. Also in more complex designs, non-parametric tests may not give proper analysis.

Features:
- It enables very few assumptions.
- It works out without using any pre-computed statistic as an estimate of parameter.
- It can be used for very small sample.
- It does not require normal distribution of the variables.
- It can be computed by very simple method.

Merits & Demerits of Non-Parametric Test:
Merits:
- It can be applied in all types of data.
- It is generally simple to understand and very easy to compute and apply.
- It has greater range of applicability.
- It does not require lengthy and laborious calculations.
- It does not need pre-computed statistics.

Demerits:

- It is often wasteful of information and less efficient.
- It sometimes pays for freedom assumptions.
- This procedure throws away information.
- This procedure has lack of power.

Differences between Parametric and Non-parametric Tests

The fundamental differences between parametric and non-parametric test are discussed in the following points:

1. A statistical test, in which specific assumptions are made about the population parameter, is known as the parametric test. A statistical test used in the case of non-parametric independent variables is called non-parametric test.

2. In the parametric test, the entire test is based on probability distribution. On the other hand, the non parametric test is distribution free test.

3. In the parametric test, the variables of interest are measured on interval or ratio level. As opposed to this in non-parametric test, the variables of interest are measured on nominal or ordinal scale.

4. In general, the parameter in parametric test is mean, while in the case of the non-parametric test it is median.

5. In the parametric test, there is complete information about the population distribution. Conversely, in the non-parametric test, there is no information about the population distribution.

6. The applicability of parametric test is for variables only, whereas non-parametric test applies to both variables and attributes.

Wilcoxon Rank Sum Test / Wilcoxon signed rank test

The t-test is the standard test for testing that the difference between population means for two paired sample is equal. If the populations are non–normal, particularly for small samples, then t-test may not be valid. The Wilcoxon Rank sum test is non-parametric test. Wilcoxon Rank sum test is used to compare the averages of two treatments/population.

That is this test is used to test the null hypothesis.

H_0: There is no significant difference between averages of two treatments against

H_1: There is significance difference between averages of two treatments.

Test procedure is to test $H_0: \mu_1 = \mu_2$ against $H_1: \mu_1 \neq \mu_2$.

Let R_1 denote sum of the ranks of the value of first sample and R_2 denote sum of the ranks of the values of the second sample.

Let R = sum of ranks for smaller sized sample.

Let n_1 = smaller sample size, Let n_2 = larger sample size.

Test statistic to be used is

$$T = \frac{(R - E(R))}{\sqrt{S_R^2}}$$

Under H_0, T has normal distribution with mean 0 and variance 1.

Critical value of above test $Z_{\alpha/2}$ such that $P[|T_{cal}| > Z_{\alpha/2}] = \alpha$

Test procedure is if $T \geq Z_{\alpha/2}$ at α % level of significance then, we reject H_0, otherwise we do not reject H_0.

Example 12: The following example gives changes in weight of control animals compared with animals given an anorexic drug. Test whether is there any effect of drug on weights of animals?

Solution:

Control animals		Drug given to animals	
Weight change (gm)	Rank	Weight change (gm)	Rank
0	9	-2	10.5
-3	9	-8	3
+9	17	+1	15
-1	12.5	-19	1
-4	7.5	-4	7.5
+3	16	-2	10.5
-1	12.5	-11	2
-5	5.5	-5	5.5
		-7	4
	Sum of ranks=94		Sum of ranks=59

Combining data for both weight change for control animals and drug treated animals is then assigned with ranks. Whenever two observations are same give same rank for both observations by taking average of ranks.

In above example we have -5 which occurs 2 times.

Therefore it has rank 5 and 6 (for next observation). Thus given 5.5 rank to both observations -5.

The test procedure is to test H_0: there is no effect of anorexic drug on the animals, against H_1: there is effect of anorexic drug on the animal.

Given that $\alpha = 0.05$ as level of significance.

Test statistic to be used is

$T = \dfrac{(R-E(R))}{\sqrt{S_R^2}}$, where n_1 = smaller sample size=8, n_2= larger sample size = 9.

R = sum of ranks for smaller sized sample = 94.

Where $E(R) = \dfrac{n_1(n_1 + n_2 + 1)}{2}$, $S_R^2 = \dfrac{n_1 n_2 (n_1 + n_2 + 1)}{12}$

$E(R) = \dfrac{n_1(n_1 + n_2 + 1)}{2} = \dfrac{8(8+9+1)}{2} = 72.$

$S_R^2 = \dfrac{n_1 n_2(n_1 + n_2 + 1)}{12} = \dfrac{8 \times 9 \times (8+9+1)}{12} = 108.$

$T = \dfrac{(R - E(R))}{\sqrt{S_R^2}} = \dfrac{(94-72)}{\sqrt{108}} = 2.12.$

Under H_0, test statistic T has standard normal distribution.

Critical value for above test =1.96 at 5% level of significance.

Test procedure to be used is if $|T| \geq Z_{\alpha/2} = 1.96$ we reject H_0 at 5% level of significance, otherwise accept H_0.

For above example T= $2.12 \geq Z_{\alpha/2} = 1.96$.

$\therefore$ Reject H_0 at 5% level of significance.

Thus there is effect of drug on animals.

Kruskal-wallis one way ANOVA :

Kruskal-wallis test is a non-parametric method for testing whether samples originate from the same distribution. It is used for comparing two or more independent samples of equal or different sample sizes. Since it is a non–parametric, the Kruskal-wallis test does not assume a normal distribution of the residuals, unlike the analogous one-way analysis of variance. However while using the Kruskal-wallis test, we do not have to make any of the assumptions of parametric test.

Therefore, the Kruskal-wallis test can be used for both continuous and ordinal level dependent variable. However, like most non-parametric tests, the Kruskal-wallis test is not as powerful as the ANOVA.

The test procedure to be used is H_0: The samples (groups) are from identical populations, against H_1: Atleast one of the samples (groups) comes from a different population than the others.

Assumptions:
We assume that the samples drawn from the population are random.
We also assume that the observations are independent of each other.
The measurement scale for the dependent variable should be at least ordinal.

Method:
1.　Rank all data from all groups together i.e. rank the data from 1 to N ignoring group membership. Assign average of the ranks to any tied values they would have received.
2.　***The test statistics is given by***:

$$H = \left[\frac{12}{N(N+1)} \sum_{I=1}^{K} \frac{T_j^2}{n_j}\right] - 3(N+1)$$

　　Where N= sum of sample size for all samples,
　　K = number of samples, T_j = sum of ranks of ith sample, n_i = size of the ith sample
3.　Find the critical x^2 value with k-1 degrees of freedom and at α =0.05 level of significance.
4.　If the critical value x^2 value is less than the H statistic, reject the H_0 that the samples are from identical population.
5.　i.e. if $H \geq x^2_{(\alpha, k-1)}$, Then reject H_0.

Example 13: Effect of Ranitidine and Omeprazole on ulcer index is evaluated in wistar rats subjected to cold restraint stress.

Ulcer index		
Serial Number	**Ranitidine 50 mg/kg**	**Omeprazole 10 mg/kg**
1	0.24	0.14
2	0.28	0.16
3	0.22	0.18
4	0.23	0.11
5	0.23	0.12
6	0.26	0.13

Determine at 5% level of significance whether there is a difference between effect of the Ranitidine and Omeprazole on ulcer index in wistar rats subjected to cold restraint stress.

Solution:

Hypothesis to be tested is H_0: there is no difference between effect of the Ranitidine and Omeprazole on ulcer index Wistar rats subjected to cold restraint stress induced ulcers, against H_1: there is a difference between effect of the Ranitidine and Omeprazole on ulcer index wistar rats subjected to cold restraint stress induced ulcers.

Since there are two data, so we have to arrange the data in ascending order of magnitude and assign appropriate ranks.

Ulcer index	0.11	0.12	0.13	0.14	0.16	0.18	0.22	0.23	0.23	0.24	0.26	0.28
Ranks	1	2	3	4	5	6	7	8.5	8.5	10	11	12

$R_1 = 21$ and $R_2 = 57$

$$\therefore H = [\frac{12}{N(N+1)} \sum_{I=1}^{K} \frac{T_j^2}{n_j}] - 3(N+1) = \frac{12}{12(12+1)}\left[\frac{R_1^2}{N_1} + \frac{R_2^2}{N_2} \right] - 3(12+1)$$

$$= \frac{12}{156}\left[\frac{21^2}{6} + \frac{57^2}{6}\right] + 3(12+1) = \frac{12}{156}[73.5 + 541.5] - 39 = 47.30769231 - 39 = 8.307692308$$

here d.f. = k-1 = 2-1 = 1

And $\alpha = 0.05$ and $x^2_{(2-1),0.05} = 3.841$

Decision criteria to be used is reject H_0 at 5% level of significance if $H > x^2_{(2-1),0.05} = 3.841$.

Since $H = 8.307692308 > x^2_{(2-1),0.05} = 3.841$.

We reject H_0 at 5% level of significance.

Therefore, there is a difference between effect of the Ranitidine and Omeprazole on ulcer index wistar rats subjected to cold restraint stress.

Friedman test

Friedman test is a non-parametric test similar to parametric repeated measures ANOVA, it is used to detect differences in treatments across multiple test attempts. The procedure involves ranking each row (or block) together, then considering the values of ranks by columns applicable to complete block designs. The Friedman test is used for one-way repeated measures analysis of variance by ranks. In its use of ranks it is similar to the Kruskal-wallis one way analysis of variance by ranks. It can also be applied for continuous data that has violated the assumptions necessary to run the one way ANOVA with repeated measures (eg .data has marked deviations from normality).

Assumptions:
- One group that is measured on three or more different occasions.
- Group is a random sample from the population.
- Your dependent variable should be measured at the ordinal or continuous level.
- Samples do not need to be normally distributed.
- Blocks are mutually independent
- Observations are ranked within blocks with no ties.
  H_0: the treatments all have identical effects, or that the sample differ in some way against H_1: the treatments do have different effects.

Method:
- Sort the data into blocks (columns).
- Rank each block separately. The smallest score should get a rank of 1.
- Sum the ranks (find total for each block).
- Calculate the test statistics.

$$F = \frac{12}{(Nk(K+1))} \sum_{i=1}^{k} R_j^2 - 3N(K+1)$$

- Find the critical F value from Friedman table at 5% level of significance.
- Compare the calculated F test statistic with critical table F value.
- Reject null hypothesis if the calculated F value is larger than critical F value.

Experimental designs

So far, we have seen that statistics is a branch of science which deals with collection, presentation, analysis and interpretation of data. This analysis and interpretation will be exact if method of analysis is correctly selected by the researchers and all underlying assumptions are satisfied. Therefore collecting and analyzing data must be carefully done with systematic planning which will give less sampling error and cost involved. Thus, we can define design of experiment as complete sequence of steps taken starting from collection of data till the analysis of results which will give less sampling error at the lowest cost.

Steps involved in experimental Design:

A statistically designed investigation involves the following basic steps:
- Make clear statement of the problem.
- Formulation of hypothesis.
- Devising the experimental technique and design.
- Decide about possible outcomes, dependent variables, response factors.
- Observe that conditions necessary for the purpose are satisfied.
- Perform the experiment.
- Observe the results.
- Make analysis and draw conclusions from the results obtained.

Basic principles of experimental design:

There are three basic principles of experimental design, viz. randomization, replication and local control.

Randomization: Randomization means process of assigning the treatments to various experimental units in purely random manner. Randomization eliminates bias in any form and it equalizes even factor of variation over which we have no control, randomization tends to produce the studying groups comparable with respect to known as well as unknown factors affecting the results and guarantees that statistical tests will have valid significance level. Thus randomization makes the test valid by making it appropriate to analyze the data.

Replication: Replication means the repetition of basic experiment that is the repetition of the treatment under investigation. By replication it is possible to average out the influence of chance or error factors on different experimental units. Thus it helps in getting more reliable results.

Local control: The process of reducing the experimental error by dividing the relatively heterogeneous area into homogeneous blocks is known as local control. The local control reduces the experimental error. It is used to make results of the experiment more efficient.

Randomization and selection of sample:

For the experiment the sample unit should be selected in a purely random manner in order to avoid personal bias to a suitable sample size. Randomization in experimental design produces the comparable groups and removes bias of the researchers in the allocation of subjects and guarantees that statistical tests will have valid significance level.

Randomization can be classified into:

1. Complete randomization
2. Blocked randomization

1. Complete randomization:

In this technique the treatments are allotted at random to the experimental units over the entire experimental duration. For selecting a sample in a group we may use techniques like unbiased coin method, random number tables or lottery method for random selection e.g. if we have to see the effectiveness of two drugs on two groups of populations A and B then by unbiased coin method we select any one group at random if head occurs and apply the first method and the second method for the other group if tail occurs.

Complete randomization is useful for homogeneous experimental data. It is used in laboratory technique, biological experiments, cookery, physics, chemistry, etc. In completely randomized design one-way analysis of variance technique is used to test significant difference between the effects of treatments. Here we have only one source of variation therefore we use technique of one way ANOVA while applying treatments on units there is no restriction on replication of treatments. However disadvantage is that it is usually suited only for small number of treatments and homogeneous experimental units.

2. Blocked randomization: If the field of experimentation is not homogenous then to control variability, field is divided into groups as blocks so that whole area in a block is relatively homogenous and treatments are applied randomly. Consider an example of administering five drugs or treatments A,B,C,D,E to 30 children. Each treatment should be replicated 4 times. Then we divide whole area into individual block (according to age group of children) and each is divided into 5 units (1,2,3,4,5) and treatments are allocated randomly to the units of a block.

Units	Block1	Block2	Block3	Block4
1	C	E	A	A
2	B	C	D	E
3	A	D	E	B
4	E	B	C	D
5	D	A	B	C

In blocked randomization, blocking produces more comparable groups and for randomization random number tables may be used.

For clinical studies following designs are used:
(i)   Completely randomized design
(ii)   Parallel design
(iii)   Crossover design
(iv)   Latin square design

Parallel designs:
Parallel designs are used to study effects of two or more drugs and to each subject only a single drug is administered. In this type of design the groups are of equal sizes, one group of subject receives formulation A and another group receives the formulation B which is to be compared with formulation A. The subjects are assigned randomly to group A or group B. The major drawback of this design is that three subjects show enormous variation in drug metabolism, excretion etc. This inter-subject variation may cause bias interpretation in the comparison of the products, due to this cross over design is preferred.

Cross over design:

In cross-over design each subject receives both formulations at different times with sufficient time gaps so that the drug is washed out of the systems. Major advantage of this method is that the inter- subject variation is reduced, thus cross over design is more sensitive than parallel design. But cross over design takes longer time due to washout period between the administrations. The cross over design for comparison of two formulations using 6 subjects is shown below:

Subject	Week 1	Week 2
1	A	B
2	B	A
3	B	A
4	A	B
5	A	B
6	B	A

Latin square design: Latin square design is a special type of crossover design for comparison of two or more than two formulations or treatments. Latin square design is used where the researchers desires to control the variation in an experiment that is related to rows and columns in the experiment. The treatments are assigned at random within rows and columns, with each treatment once per row and once per column. There are equal numbers of rows, columns, and treatments. It is useful where the experimenter desires to control variation in two different directions. The design is balanced and consist of N*N arrays, where N is number of formulations or subjects or treatments.

Latin squares designs for comparing 2, 3, and 4 formulations are shown below.

2 × 2 Latin square

Subject	First week	Second week
1	A	B
2	B	A

3 × 3 Latin square

Subject	First week	Second week	Third week
1	A	B	C
2	B	C	A
3	C	A	B

4 × 4 Latin square

Subject	First week	Second week	Third week	Fourth week
1	A	B	C	D
2	B	C	D	A
3	C	D	A	B
4	D	A	B	C

Where A, B, C and D are formulations or treatments. In case of three or four formulations for comparison, viz is not possible to use crossover design. Since analysis becomes more complicated. In such case balanced incomplete block design is used. In this design each formulation or treatments occurs the same number of times and every pair of formulations or treatments occurs together in the same number of subjects. Balanced incomplete block design for comparing four formulations or treatments is given in table below:

Subject	First	Second
1	B	A
2	B	C
3	D	B
4	A	B
5	A	C
6	D	C
7	C	A
8	C	D
9	A	D
10	B	D
11	C	B
12	D	A

Thus in this design, inter subject variability is removed giving at least two formulations to each subject.

Note: The above test can be performed using statistical software like SAS, R, SPSS, etc.

Following tables shows the list of statistical softwares which are available for the statistical analysis:

Name of the software	Description
Scipy (statsmodel)	It is an open source statistical package. It performs tests like non-parametric statistics, ANOVA, GLM, time series, etc.
R software	It is an open source statistical package. It is a free implementation of the S language. It can perform all kind of statistical test. Both parametric and non-parametric.
GraphPad InStat	It is a proprietary statistical package. Very simple with lots of guidance and explanations. But it does not have analytical features for analysis of Two-way ANOVA.
GraphPad Prism	It is a proprietary statistical package. Very simple with lots of guidance and explanations. Biostatistics and nonlinear regression with clear explanations.
SPSS	It is a proprietary statistical package. It can perform all type of tests like Cross tabulation, frequencies, t-test, ANOVA, Correlation, Non-parametric tests, etc.
MATLAB	It is a proprietary statistical package. It can perform both parametric and non-parametric tests.
SAS	It is a proprietary statistical package. SAS provides a graphical point-and-click user interface for non-technical users and more advanced options through the SAS programming language. It can perform all type of statistical analysis and hence used widely.
Stats Direct	It is a proprietary statistical package. It can perform parametric tests but does not perform non parametric test.

Although there are many softwares available, most commonly used softwares in the field of pharmacy are SAS, SPSS, GraphPad Instat, GraphPad prism etc.

References:

1. Gupta S.C. and Kapoor V.K.: Fundamentals of mathematical statistics 10th edition, New delhi, S. Chand and company Ltd. pages; 2.1-18.64.

2. Daniel W.W: Applied non parametric statistics 1st edition, Boston-Houghton Miffin company, pages: 16-50.

3. Vijay.K.Rohatgi, A.K.Ehsanessaleh M.D., An introduction to probability and statistics, John Wiley and Sons, 2nd edition pages 354-391.

4. Kruskal W.H. and Wallis W.A.,1952, "Use of ranks in one criterion analysis of variance", Jour. Amer. Statist. Assoc, 47, pages 583.

5. Das, M.N. and Giri,N.C.,1979, Design and Analysis of Experiments, Wiley Eastern Pvt. Ltd. pages 126-144.

6. Lehmann E.L and Romano Joseph P., 2005, Testing statistical hypothesis 3rd edition, Springer text pages 110-276.

7. J.D.Gibbons and S. Chakrabati: Non parametric statistical inference 3rd edition, revised and expanded pages 288-307, 386-396.

8. Douglas.C.Montgomery Design and analysis of experiment, john wiley and sons inc 1997 4th edition. pages 1-20,60-125,126-144.

9. Kshirsagar A.M. A course in linear models, Marcel Dekker inc 1983.pages 161-309,377-3.

ANNEXURE

The animals are housed in opaque polypropylene cages (28 × 21 × 14 cm) and maintained in temperature and humidity-controlled holding facility 25 ± 2°C under 12:12 h light/dark cycle (07:00–14:00 h). All animals are provided food with free access to rodent chow and purified drinking water.

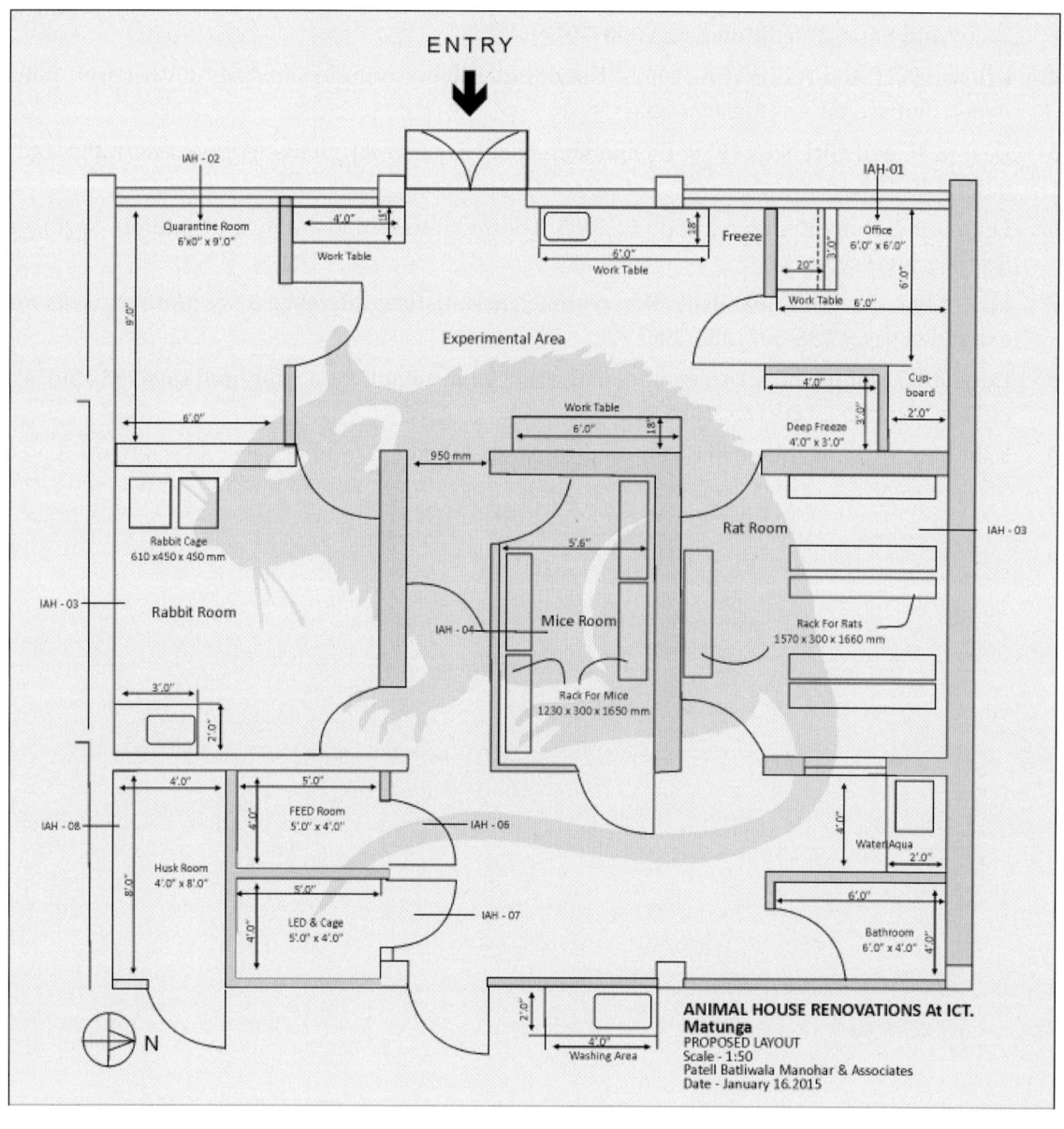

INSTITUTIONAL ANIMAL ETHICS COMMITTEE / BOARD

"Institutional Animals Ethics Committee" (IAEC) is a body comprising of a group of persons recognized and registered by the Committee for the purpose of control and supervision of experiments on animals (CPCSEA) performed in educational / research institution.

IAEC reviews and approves all types of research proposals involving small animal experimentation before the initiation of the study. For experimentation on large animals, the project is required to be forwarded to CPCSEA in prescribed format with recommendation of IAEC. IAEC is required to monitor the research progressthrough periodic reports throughout the study and after the completion of research project. The committee has to ensure compliance with all regulatory requirements, applicable rules, guidelines and laws.

Composition of IAEC shall include eight members as follows:

1. A biological scientist,
2. Two scientists from different biological disciplines,
3. A veterinarian involved in the care of animals,
4. Scientist in charge of animal's facility of the establishment concerned,
5. A scientist from, outside the institute,
6. A non scientific socially aware member and
7. A nominee of CPCSEA.

NOTES

NOTES

NOTES